The MYSTERY of JOYFUL SEX

More Than 300 Ways of Erotic and Intimate Techniques

LAURA SCOTT

Order this book online at www.trafford.com
or email orders@trafford.com

Most Trafford titles are also available at major online book retailers.

Printed in the United States of America.

ISBN: 978-1-4669-1761-3 (sc)
ISBN: 978-1-4669-1763-7 (hc)
ISBN: 978-1-4669-1762-0 (e)

Library of Congress Control Number: 2012903221

Trafford rev. 08/29/2012

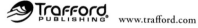 www.trafford.com

North America & international
toll-free: 1 888 232 4444 (USA & Canada)
phone: 250 383 6864 ♦ fax: 812 355 4082

This book was created thanks to the efforts of numerous people. Those individuals include girls working in massage parlors as well as experienced, mature women who really understand sex and its importance to a successful relationship. Thanks to the cooperation of those persons, we can look at intimacy through the eyes of women of diverse ages, which only makes this text that much more appealing.

CONTENTS

Part 3
Enjoy Your Femininity

Part 4
Erotic Games

PREFACE

My experience in various massage parlors, including those that offer intimate massage as a "form of therapy", has convinced me of the great importance of such procedure and the obvious demand of that service. I can attest without doubt that the demand is on the rise.

There are many reasons for such a great interest in intimate massage, the leading ones being:

- The increase in sexual problems.
- The expectation of great sexual ability from a partner.
- Sexual satisfaction through massage, especially for those who do not have a partner, and the number of single individuals is steadily increasing. In those cases, intimate massage is an alternative to a one-night stand. This method (non-penetrating activity) guarantees safety from contracting an STD in this age and offers an opportunity for releasing one's sexual tension.
- Reaching a state of full relaxation during an intimate encounter without the necessity of concentrating on one's partner, which is unavoidable in a relationship. Partners expect reciprocation, which in turn may rule

out relaxation. Besides, massage, including its intimate form, is an art that requires at least some experience so relaxation can be achieved.

- To discover one's sexual potential.
- To feel great! The human body produces endorphins, which are responsible for well-being, and they are released during prolonged arousal. Studies(1) also show that sex in moderation has a positive influence on the immune system. These findings also apply to intimate massage*. Let us not forget the role of touch itself and its healing properties (see Chapter 3).
- To check one's sexual potential. This reason relates especially to men, who would like to fully know their sexual abilities and thus confirm, for example, the quality of their erection, its duration, or perhaps the quantity of ejaculations in a given amount of time.
- When it comes to women, breast examination and massage of breasts.
- Intimate massage can help awaken a woman's sexual potential through touch, especially for those women who have problems climaxing.

The increase of people suffering from sexual inadequacies in the past few decades is great. These individuals include those whose sexual problems are a direct result of other maladies caused in large part by air and water contamination; the use of chemicals in food production and storage; unsanitary living conditions; lack of exercise; stress; and unhealthy eating habits. All those factors which are very closely connected with our rapid technological advancement have a significant negative effect on our health.

Intimate massage enables us to uncover our sexual potential. Using different techniques helps us determine what stimulates our sex drives. Sometimes such revelation can be very unexpected. The basis of a successful sexual relationship is the knowledge of your and your partner's bodies and their reactions to stimulants.

Teaching and demonstrating the classical version of the intimate massage are functions of a massage parlor. It has become quite popular, and not only for young people. Fascination with the other sex's anatomy and physiology of the intimate parts has drawn people of all ages. It appears that many of us still have a lot to learn about intimacy, and we are ready to embark on that journey. It is important to know about these things because the lack of this knowledge often causes improper stimulation of a partner, which may lead to uncomfortable situations.

Another variable responsible for the increase of necessity of massage parlors, including intimate massage, is young individuals who decide to not engage in long-term relationships and whose source of sexual satisfaction is intimate massage. Instead of involving themselves in risky short-term sexual encounters with strangers, they choose a safer alternative. People who are between relationships or have separated while working out their problems and those who have decided not to start having intercourse yet are in a similar situation. In reality, these are individuals who use this type of massage as a substitute for sex. While AIDS is still a realistic threat, such a solution definitely makes sense.

Intimate massage can also be an alternative to becoming sexually active at a very young age(2), which seems to be more and more common these days. Oftentimes sheer curiosity and not actual sexual excitement makes young people, especially girls, decide to experiment with sex. This curiosity in many cases turns into a desire to see a penis, to touch it, to see an erection and an ejaculation. This becomes so interesting to them they agree to have intercourse, not because they desire it, but because they want to satisfy their curiosity about their partner's body. It is only natural to be curious about the sexual reactions of the opposite sex, but learning about them does not have to be synonymous with intercourse. One of the goals of massage parlors is to help young people in this area, although they are not limited to just that. Another mission is to provide information on how to have safe sex and how to prevent pregnancies.

The Mystery of Joyful Sex promotes healthy, safe, and fun sexual experiences, especially in the form of intimate massage. It also suggests ways to bring more excitement into the bedroom through erotic games and foreplay. Many of those offers not only provide pleasure, but they often also have a self healing effect. They are a source of satisfaction and great intimacy for men and women. Intimate massage may be a "form of therapy" for those who have become addicted not only to sex. It can help overcome addictions. (3) Having sex just to have sex is pointless. After all, its purpose is to attain joy from being with one's partner, to relax, to reach ecstasy, and to feel great, as well as to learn and accept your and your partner's needs.

Unfortunately, these goals seem to lose importance as the level of sexual attraction decreases in a relationship. Intimate and erotic massage can help realize the importance of these values even for those partners who are bored with each other. Instead of changing partners, it is worth giving intimate massage a shot.

The following was written by a steady client of a massage parlor in response to my questionnaire about her experiences: "Intimate massage is a great experience that can replace sexual intercourse as well as oral sex, which is considered by many men as the most exciting form of sexual experience. Not all women, especially those who are just beginning their sexual journey, are ready for oral sex, and intercourse isn't always possible for them. A good alternative is, of course, intimate massage. A correctly performed massage can be an awesome experience, which can be hard to believe if you haven't experienced it before. It can be a great way to complement your sex life."

INTRODUCTION

This book is devoted to three issues: the joy of sex, intimate massage, and erotic games and foreplay. The keystone is intimate touch. Its function cannot be overestimated, not only in its relation to sex but also to health, personal well-being, cheerfulness, life energy, etc. Its most evident role is in intimate massage. Of course things are different between people dear to one another and strangers. In the first instance, intimate massage can be a prelude to sex, while in the second case it is just a service performed for a specific purpose. This publication is intended as much for the single audience as for couples. This is why sex and massage are intertwined in this book. However, it does not mean I am encouraging sexual intercourse at the end of a massage, unless of course it is a result of the partners' closeness and spontaneity.

While working in an intimate massage parlor, I noticed its very important purpose. The therapeutic effects depend on the masseur's or masseuse's skills (and the patient's discipline), not on the institution. On the other hand, the existence of such places surely allows this form of "therapy" and relaxation to become more common.

So what is this book about? It is not a medical publication or a textbook containing precise rules of conduct. Its purpose is to be more of a guide rather than a set of regulations. This publication shows the outstanding role of intimate massage for our health and well being. There is no overstatement using the term "*therapeutic intimate massage*" for this special kind of massage because its proper use leads to the production of excess amount of endorphins, which affect our mood. This mechanism of our brain activity was described in *Sexual Healing* by Barbara Keesling, PhD.

It turns out that the same results can be achieved during intimate massage. So this is why more than three hundred types and methods of erotic and intimate touch have been used throughout the book. There is not the point to check all of them but to choose reasonable quantity corresponding to our temperament. Also, to avoid monotony.

There is no wrong way to have consensual adult sex (or intimate massage), and the quality of the experience is measured by the level of satisfaction of both partners. Problems arise when there is little or no satisfaction. The cause of continually diminishing sexual pleasure vary from person to person. For example, people in long-term relationships often tend to fall into a routine, where the bedroom becomes "sexual fast food," so to speak—come in, satisfy the hunger, get out—which in the long run can be as harmful as fast food itself.

Wildly believed stereotypes are often another reason for the lack of or lessened pleasure during intercourse. Some of these stereotypes have become so common that nobody questions their validity. For example, millions of men are convinced that their unsuccessful love lives would improve only if they had a larger penis, while their women are sure that the only way to become the ideal lover is to act like a porn star. In many cases, both genders agree that the only gauge of sexual satisfaction is an orgasm. Other issues, such as getting to know each other better, exploring new territories, enjoying a lover's tender touch, or just being close to one another take second place. Consequently, making love becomes something purely mechanical, like a list of tasks that need to be accomplished in order to feel a sense of fulfillment. It becomes yet another chore. Instead of bringing people closer together it splits them apart, changing an intimate encounter into an exchange of services. This book will show that sex is so much more than that—it is an art form of its own. What counts in any form of art aside from the end result is the creative process and the tools used throughout it, the most essential being imagination.

Remember that by taking time to read this book there is nothing to lose, except a conventional outlook on sexuality, and there is so much to gain. Satisfaction in the bedroom is, after all, synonymous with satisfaction from life. *In the bedroom,* in this case, means not only traditional sex but intimate and erotic massage, as well as any erotic games and foreplay. These elements of intimate relationships produce intense pleasure, without which life would just not be as satisfying.

DISCLAIMER

It should be noted that all information in this book, while being useful in dealing with a variety of sexual ailments, and serving as a guide to healthy and enjoyable intimate relations, should not be treated as a method of either diagnosing, treating or curing any medical conditions. All the methods described in the book were gathered solely for information purposes and they should not substitute medical advice from licensed medical professionals. Just like with any kind of physical activity, each individual might be affected in a different way by the methods described. Before performing any activities listed in the book, one should consult a physician or other licensed medical professional.

CHAPTER 1

For Those Who Want to Give a Massage

When I started working in an intimate massage parlor, I was convinced my work would consist of, more or less, the same activities that a woman normally engages in during foreplay with a man—meaning sexually exciting him by stimulating his penis with her hand. The only difference between such massage and intercourse—in my and my friends' opinions (with whom I have spent countless hours discussing this and similar topics)—is that during intercourse, a man usually reaches an orgasm inside the woman, while during a massage the climactic moment is external, stimulated solely by the hand of the masseuse. The work seemed easy and attractive, in addition to being well paying.

I quickly realized, after my friends and I shared our intimate experiences with the opposite sex with each other, how little I knew about sex, men's sexual needs, their different sexual reactions, or even erotic "tricks" and different techniques of stimulating the penis. Thus, I concluded that working in an intimate massage parlor would enable me to learn those arcana, which I considered extremely beneficial to my intimate relations with men. I knew how much men valued women's knowledge about sex, but I did not know what this knowledge consisted of. My friends had a similar dilemma—we all wanted to be adults, have sex, and impress our peers with that fact, but we did not really know much about it.

And so, with much hope I began working in the intimate massage parlor, convinced that my job would be easy, enjoyable, and financially satisfying. I have to attest that I was not wrong, except for a few reservations. I quickly grasped that it was not a game but real, responsible work, which required much knowledge and experience, people skills, sensitivity, a sense of humor, and the ability to establish trust between my clients and me. Trust, the guarantee of full discretion, and a professional approach to each patient* and his problems are the basis of success of the "therapy" and the career.

I comprehended, only after some time, how stressed out the men who come in for therapeutic intimate massage can be. Not only do they suffer from sexual dysfunctions (which is stressful enough), they have additional stress as a result of being completely naked in the presence of a strange woman. Diminished sexual capability, or lack of one, causes men to be quite sensitive and/or irritable. This is why a masseuse must be conscientious about her every word and reaction. Even though a reaction can be a normal and natural behavior, it may be misinterpreted by the patient. Gaining the patient's trust is at least half the battle in curing their sexual dysfunctions. Many patients become regular guests of our massage parlor, even after they reach full sexual well being and end up in healthy, meaningful relationships because it is the only place where they feel truly mentally and physically relaxed. Only here they do not have to be at their best or prove anything to themselves or their partners, especially their sexual abilities. We realize their reactions are natural—and we treat them in such way. For example, if a man suffers from premature ejaculation, it does not necessarily mean he has a sexual inadequacy. The reason may be his young age, his vast sexual needs, or the lack of a permanent partner. Also, erectile dysfunction in a stressful situation is a normal reaction of the body. Suspecting a man of a disorder in such a situation may, in fact, through the power of suggestion, drive him to one. Men are sensitive about their manhood, and any failure in their intimate lives equals a national disaster.

Before I started working in the parlor, I was told that regardless of my experience in the field, I had to complete an intimate massage course. My instructor was a career masseuse who was not only an excellent professional in her field but had a great, natural ability for sharing her knowledge and skills. I strongly encourage those interested in learning the art of intimate massage to take such a course and have the chance to be instructed by an expert, someone who has, aside from knowledge and experience, the gift of conveying that information to others. Unfortunately, not all of us have that quality—and this is where this book comes in handy.

During my first session of the course, my instructor said, "You will never be a good intimate massage therapist—and such work will only be troublesome to you—if you do not like playing with a penis, if you only fondle it in order to receive pleasure in return. If such is the case, you should look for a different job." (The same goes for men who want to practice "intimate massage therapy" for women but expect reciprocation of services.)

I was always fascinated by the penis. I love to feel it in my hand—its throbbing, the growth of an erection caused by my touch, its hardness. I know I make that happen and draw pleasure and strength from that fact. It amazes me that I can have such control over men—who are strong and physically fit—by appropriately taking care of them. I've noticed that playing with a penis is not only beneficial to men—I always felt great, both physically and mentally, afterward. The more I fondled and caressed it, the more powerful I felt. With time I found out that this feeling of power is simply the energy awakened in a man by arousing him and then transferred to the woman through physical contact. This physical contact could be of any kind and does not necessarily have to be intercourse—which, by the way, is "against the law" in intimate massage parlors (it is only allowed in sex therapy, where intercourse is a form of healing).

Anna, my instructor, explained that the work of an intimate massage specialist has nothing to do with the work of a prostitute. Prostitutes offer their bodies and services in return for money to pleasure their clients and satisfy their sexual needs. The goal of intimate massage is to treat ailments, not only those of an intimate nature but including those that manifest themselves as sexual disorders, and many others.

To give you an example, Anna talked about the many reasons for erectile dysfunction. She said there does not have to be anything wrong with the penis itself; instead, the man might be stressed out, overworked, undernourished, or perhaps he lost interest in his partner. The reasons are numerous, but the important thing is that our services enable them to feel self-confident, relaxed, and refreshed while we gain a regular customer.

Another difference between the work of an intimate masseuse and the work of a prostitute is that the type of treatment a man receives in our parlors is decided by a doctor or masseuse and not by the customer. To us, that person is a patient seeking help, not someone expecting to satisfy their erotic fantasies. This is the key difference and it must be remembered at all times while at work. The work of a therapist in an intimate massage parlor is not unlike the work of a nurse, and just because it deals with the intimate side of life, it does not change that fact. I feel that my work is very important because sexual problems are extremely irritating for anyone experiencing them. Since sex is an important part of life we should not disregard the problems associated with it.

The need of specialized intimate massage parlors should now be obvious to those who were unsure of their necessity. They are just like any of the other massage parlors that thrive in our communities. People go there to relieve pain, stress, and anxiety. They go there to get treated, get helped, and get better. And since massage is good for the whole body, it is a logical conclusion that it is good for its intimate parts. To think otherwise is to label different body parts as "good" and "bad," as "holy" and "unholy." The negative effects of such a point of view are so obvious, it's astonishing how many followers it still has.

Modern literature that deals with sexual problems tells us that the basics of a successful "therapy" are the exercises involving intimate massage with another person. Of course it is not enough to just know the techniques of intimate massage for healing someone. There are other criteria, such as trust, the patient's mood during a session, the ability to fully relax, the acceptance of one's body and its reactions, overall self-confidence, patience, etc. Partners are not always able to provide all those elements, no matter how much they care about one another. Other times the patient does not want to reveal the problem to someone close to him but wants to seek help from a complete stranger. He prefers to appear healthy and sexually able to his partner.

And what about those who are not in relationship, or those who avoid them because of their sexual inadequacies? Should they not have the means for getting better and enjoying a human connection?

Of course the act of intercourse is not everything. A conversation, being with the other person, and mutual caressing are important. Touch itself has a great significance in the healing process. Furthermore, endorphins (the "feel good" hormone, amongst other things—but more on endorphins later in the book), play an important role in our bodies. They are released approximately an hour after the start of sexual stimulation.

Other research(4) indicates that being sexually active twice a week has a positive effect on the immune system. If anyone still doubts the purpose of the existence of intimate massage parlors, they should try to solve the dilemma of a frustrated woman who cannot reach an orgasm because of an underdeveloped G-spot. In such a case, reaching an orgasm is only possible through regular and skillful stimulation. It is not enough to diagnose the ailment; it still has to be treated—in this instance by intimate massage. Should that woman give up the wonderful experience of an orgasm because she does not have a partner or he is not patient and understanding enough? Of course not, especially since an orgasm does not just feel good, it is good for the body and has a positive effect on its functions.

Same goes for male impotence. Sometimes the problem can be quickly solved by changing the technique of stimulation or combining a few. Other times the problem will have a deeper cause and thus require a different approach. This is why it takes a qualified, competent specialist* to diagnose the problem. It is unlikely that a wife or lover will be able to do so without prior training. A call girl is not going to be much help either.

If anyone still has doubts regarding this form of "therapy", they should try out its effectiveness for themselves. After an hour with a professional masseuse no one should fail to see the sense of intimate massage and the role it plays in peoples' health and general well being.

Anna warned me several times to make sure I know that this type of work can be satisfying and profitable—under the condition that I will be determined to thoroughly learn the theory of intimate massage and be able to correctly apply it in reality. "It is a form of massage," she reminded me, "not a game with a patient's body."

Unfortunately, many women, young and mature, think otherwise. It is not uncommon to find such a mindset in some massage parlors (for men). The philosophy, as well as practice of medicinal intimate massage, does not share this misconception. A future massage therapist must pass an exam upon the completion of the course. In addition, it is the therapist's duty to keep up with the latest studies and to take additional courses to sharpen his or her skills.

Before a new masseuse is able to start a job, she must sign a non-disclosure agreement, which ensures, under a heavy monetary penalty, the confidentiality of the patients' information. It means the therapist must keep confidential the information entrusted to her by her patients, even after she no longer works in her profession. The patients' trust in the therapist and the therapist's loyalty toward the patients are crucial factors in the healing process. A successful therapy oftentimes depends upon fully opening up to a therapist. If at any time a patient has even the slightest suspicion of a breach of confidentiality, the patient can develop a block—which can, in turn, stop or even reverse the progress made in therapy, even to the point of making the problem worse. It is extremely important to remember that sexual ailments are, by nature, a very sensitive subject and that it is men who are usually oversensitive about them. There just is no room for any suspicion that a third party can find out any of their private information.

From the beginning, I was reminded to take every patient and their problems seriously, even those whose issues seem to be figments of their imagination. If someone does not feel well, but the problem cannot be diagnosed, it still does not change the fact that something is not right with that person. The subjective experience of each person is what counts. Take this case as an example: a series of tests indicate that a man is healthy, yet he feels unhappy because of—in his opinion—an incomplete erection. It is useless to try to persuade him not to worry; instead, it is better to find an appropriate exercise that will help him realize he is perfectly fine.

One more important thing was emphasized during the preparatory course: the ability to accept each person just the way he or she is. Not every man is Apollo and not every woman is Venus. Well, maybe in Hollywood, but not in real life, of course, and that is normal. It is obvious that since every person has anatomical differences, his or her intimate areas are not identical either. Even if something is surprisingly strange or "funny" to us as therapists, we have to make sure to not make that apparent to the patient. The patient has to be comfortable and have a feeling of acceptance by the therapist. Penis size and the speed of the reaction to outside stimuli are touchy subjects for many men, and a reckless word or gesture may be misinterpreted as an allusion to their manhood. It is a complicated matter because one man will think that an erection should occur the moment he sees a naked woman, considering it a sign of health, while another will think that a quick erection is jumping the gun and will be afraid of a tendency toward premature ejaculation.

I have had many cases where a man came in for treatment because he was convinced he could not "get it up" any more, yet he showed signs of arousal only moments after the start of the intimate examination. As I have stated before, men are extremely sensitive when it comes to their sexual abilities. If a partner cannot create the right mood or fails to stimulate him correctly, if they fight constantly or she humiliates him (not necessarily in bed, but just throughout the day), then he might not be able to get aroused, convincing himself that there is something wrong with him. In many cases this can be easily reversed if his partner gives him a boost of confidence and shows him some affection, which, combined with the proper stimulation, will give him the psychological comfort necessary to regain his usual abilities, and of course the joy of life as well.

CHAPTER 2

More than Words: Sensual Massage and Other Pleasures

The statement "sex sells" is nothing new in today's world. Sex is used to market products in a variety of different industries—from automobiles to magazines and even groceries. It captures the customers' attention by appealing to their sense of sight. In effect, the human body is primarily associated with being looked at and not as much with being touched, much to our disadvantage. We are able to become aroused at the sight of an attractive body, but we can fully interact with that person only through touching and caressing—the most primal yet underestimated forms of communication. It seems that for many people this sort of intimacy is awkward, even inappropriate, so they limit themselves to cold, calculated intercourse deprived of any real closeness. Even if they master the most imaginative sexual positions and techniques possible, they are missing an element, sensuality, without which discussing sex in its complete form is impossible.

Sexuality and sensuality are like two spices that must be added to a "meal called life" in order to make it taste right. Unfortunately, as already mentioned in the introduction, many individuals too often give up a gourmet dish for fast food. Some individuals get stuck in the monotony of the unexplored bedroom, believing that's just the way it is, or decide to change partners, thinking it will help them find that long-lost excitement. This is how the logic of the vicious cycle of being unfulfilled is born.

Those people give up their happiness or look for it in the wrong places without realizing that it is literally at their fingertips. Touch is often taken for granted, while that very sense enables people to overstep the boundaries set forth by their minds and actually open up to their partners, therefore creating a successful, happy, and long-lasting relationship. Everyone can reach their partners' emotional and spiritual realms and show them, through physical contact, how much they mean to them. Finally, they can feel better physically themselves, which promotes their mental well being and health in general.

Massage is one of the oldest yet simplest forms of healing known to mankind. It is recognized as a great type of therapy for many health issues, including stress-related, nervous, and emotional problems. The use of massage was widespread throughout and important to many Eastern cultures for a long time. Doctors from those regions have been using massage for healing purposes, as well as preventative care, for a few thousand years now. Some of the ancient Chinese, Egyptian, and Hindu writings of medical practices describe different forms of massage.

Massage helps a person find inner peace, which in turn can have a soothing effect on others. According to many therapists**(5)**, massage can bring people closer together and improve their emotional contact as well as their erotic lives.

What is massage? It is a form of touching based on methodical movements, which are applied to get certain results. Another good, simple way to look at it is that massage is a form of physical contact between people, during which a person's hands touch another person's skin. This natural procedure can have healing or recreational applications. It is believed that the most important element of massage is the transfer of energy among people.

According to some experts, touch is the first sense that develops in the womb(6). They claim that this sense is a fundamental human need, without which we cannot exist. Thus we cannot underestimate the role of touch in our lives. A good example is a study conducted on a group of infants that were split into two groups. One group was exposed to more touch than the other, and the results clearly showed a difference. Those infants who received more physical interaction developed faster than those who had less.

One should familiarize herself with a few different kinds of massages, which are used in my line of work:

- Relaxing massage
- Erotic (sensual) massage
- Intimate-erotic massage
- Relaxing-intimate massage or classic intimate massage
- Healing-intimate massage

We will briefly discuss these types of massage because some basic knowledge is needed; however, since the focus of this book is intimate massage, we will not go into much detail.

Relaxing massage

The purpose of a relaxing massage is, as the name indicates, to relax. It can serve as an introduction to an erotic or intimate massage. It can be foreplay to sex, or it can just be what it is—a relaxing massage. However, in most cases it is the first step to intimate, erotic, and healing massages. It can be alternately used with intimate massage to control the level of arousal. If the arousal is too high during an intimate massage, it is better to switch to relaxing massage than to stop massaging altogether. This massage, unlike the other kinds, does not require a close bond or intimacy between partners. As its name suggests, this massage is used to fight stress and other ailments associated with it, such as headaches, backaches, problems with concentrating, depression, and general fatigue. It is possible to do all these things through stimulation of muscles, skin, and circulation, which affect the nervous system responsible for neutralizing the negative effects of stress, thus releasing muscle tension; regulating the heartbeat, blood flow, and pressure; as well as helping combat insomnia or sleeplessness. The buildup of muscular, nervous, and psychological tension is first decreased and then eliminated, leading to full relaxation. This state of relaxation is achieved through gentle, slow, calm, rhythmic movements of the masseuse's hands. Relaxing massage is great for everyone regardless of age, sex, or health problems.

Erotic (sensual) massage

This type of massage requires much more emotional involvement from both partners. Key elements of this massage are mutual trust, plenty of time, and an ability to calm down. This type of massage is not recommended for one-night stands. Different forms of this massage are considered foreplay. Oftentimes erotic massage is mistaken with intimate massage, but the difference is fundamental. Intimate massage can be the substitute for intercourse while erotic massage cannot.

Erotic massage should be performed in an intimate setting with no disturbances. Plenty of time is essential as well, so it is best to do this after all daily responsibilities have been completed.

The place should be roomy and comfortable. It is recommended to put a mattress directly on the floor, as a bed might be too soft for certain parts of the massage that require more strength.

The topic of this book is intimate massage, which is often incorrectly mistaken for erotic massage. There is, however, a big and fundamental difference between the two. Erotic massage can, in fact, serve as an introduction to intimate massage; it focuses on erogenous areas of the body such as the ears, the back, and the buttocks but not the reproductive organs, which belong to the domain of intimate massage.

The purpose of erotic massage is to cause sexual arousal in one's partner. It can lead to intercourse, but that does not have to be the goal. For example, a massage used to sensitize breasts is purely a sensual massage. However, in most cases, erotic massage is followed by intimate massage and sex. The use of intimate massage for healing purposes, through stimulation of intimate areas, does not have to end with the release of sexual tension. Oftentimes it does not, especially if the purpose of the procedure is to reach and maintain a high level of arousal for a given period of time. If the goal is reached, only then is an orgasm allowed. However, if the goal is to awaken someone's sexuality, then the massage does not have to lead to an orgasm. The outcome of the massage depends upon each individual case.

As I have mentioned, erotic massage is supposed to cause sexual arousal, which is why it focuses on respective parts of the body known as the erogenous zones, which exclude the reproductive organs. Erogenous areas have an exceptionally great erotic potential, and their stimulation leads to sexual arousal. More on this topic in later chapters.

The difference between relaxing massage and erotic massage is that during an erotic massage, one focuses on the erogenous zones, while during a relaxing massage one usually avoids them. The use of relaxing touch is to create a feeling of subtle pleasure but not sexual arousal. However, a person can become aroused through relaxing massage unintentionally because everyone is different. The human body is sensitive to touch, and the threshold of sensitivity on different body parts may be different for everyone. We all have erogenous areas of the body, but the location of those spots may vary slightly from person to person. This is why one must not only know the definition of erogenous areas but also be able to apply it in practice. It is important in my line of work because while performing a relaxing massage, I may notice a patient's excitement, and my patient may be surprised to experience sexual arousal, even though it theoretically should not have happened. In such cases, it is crucial to remember individual circumstances instead of jumping to conclusions and accusing one another of ignoble intentions. It is a good idea for a patient to communicate with his therapist and let her know how sensitive his body is or the type of reactions he is prone to.

I would like to reiterate the difference between intimate and erotic massage. In a nutshell, intimate massage includes the massage of intimate areas (the vulva for women and the penis and testicles for men) while erotic massage does not.

An orgasm is not the goal of erotic massage, but it is possible for one to occur. It does not mean that one crossed the boundary between erotic and intimate massage. What it does mean is that most likely the person receiving the massage is very sensitive to touch (and it is possible the masseuse is quite skilled as well).

Breast massage in most cases is considered to be erotic massage, but in some women those areas are so sensitive that their stimulation may cause an orgasm.

Side note

The round shape of breasts is primarily a sexual and not a nurturing function. Take for example monkeys who are flat-chested yet are able to breastfeed. In humans the amount of milk created by a woman is not dependant upon her breast size.

These are the things patients most often expect from an erotic massage:

- pleasure from massaging the erogenous zones
- the experience of something new (the use of different accessories for the massage, e.g., water, hair, or breasts)
- to check the effectiveness of massage
- the massage of a specific body part, usually not stimulated in a classic massage, but which is pleasurable to the patient
- to firm the bosom* (see "Subconsciousness")
- to see if erotic massage can lead to orgasm
- to prepare for an intimate moment with one's partner. The patient may worry about not satisfying his partner because of a lack of arousal.
- as an introduction to intimate massage

Erotic-intimate massage

This type of massage has the characteristics of an erotic massage but can also include the massage of intimate areas of the body. It does not mean it is just an erotic massage culminated with masturbation. It is a massage during which the masseuse takes turns using the two forms of massage or uses them simultaneously, in which case one hand stimulates an erogenous area, while the other—an intimate one.

Intimate massage

Intimate massage is not just an act of masturbating someone else. The purpose of masturbation is to reach orgasm. An orgasm can and often is achieved during an intimate massage; however, its basis is a specific technique. The destination is not as important as the means itself. So what is an intimate massage? Put simply, it is a massage of intimate areas, which affects the whole body. It can have a relaxing as well as healing effect, depending on the goal.

Intimate massage is essentially the caressing of the genitals and their neighboring areas. For men, that is the penis and testicles but also the crotch and groin. The sensitivity of the member is comparable to the sensitivity of the clitoris, but the mechanics of intimate massage differ in both sexes. Intimate massage of the penis can be initiated without previously engaging in erotic massage, while the vagina requires some foreplay in the form of massage of the erogenous areas. It is a common misconception that the massage of a penis has to be firm, uninterrupted, and decisive. It is a big mistake because if a man is very aroused, such massage will end with an ejaculation too fast, and that is not the purpose of intimate massage. Of course an orgasm can be achieved as a result of intimate massage, but it should not happen accidentally; it should be controlled—and ejaculation should take place only when desired. However, there are instances when a man expects and wants a firm grip on his penis and quick, decisive movements of a woman's hand.

An extremely sensitive spot is the *frenulum of prepuce of the penis.* * This area is where the skin, which begins in the crotch and runs up the penis including the testes, meets the glans penis. It is visible when the foreskin is retracted (it is best seen when a man is lying on his back with an erection). The frenulum can be stimulated by rubbing it directly or through the foreskin. The glans, commonly known as the head is the top of the member and is a very sensitive body part. It requires much caution, especially when the foreskin is pulled back. This is why lube is recommended before any stimulation of the head is begun. One should also pay attention to the tip where the urethral opening is located.

The purpose of intimate massage

The goal of intimate massage is not just pleasure: it is meant to enhance health and general well being, to increase arousal, to heal many ailments (not only related to sex), and as a preventative measure. Here is a list of a few of the numerous benefits of intimate massage:

- inner peace
- better mood
- deeper state of relaxation
- increased libido
- increased sexual potency
- better health (when used regularly for a longer period of time)

• better circulation

Therapeutic intimate massage is the most common of massages used in therapeutic intimate massage parlors, but it is not the only one. The other kinds are used mostly to complement it. There are instances where intimate massage is not necessary, and all that is needed is a relaxing or erotic massage. In most cases, those two forms of massage serve as an introduction to intimate massage or are used in conjunction with it. Going back and forth among the different kinds of massages has good reasons, for example, to prevent excessive arousal if it is not recommended for therapeutic purposes.

Therefore, we may differentiate between relaxing-intimate massage and healing-intimate massage.

Relaxing-intimate massage

It is a form of intimate massage and its purpose is sexual pleasure, but it is unlike regular caressing because it is based on repetition, certain motions, certain pressure of the grasp, and similar factors. It can be pleasure in itself or can be used as a form of foreplay, but its most important attribute is the relaxation it provides. Mutual exploration of intimate massage is the key to wonderful experiences. If one is not sure what satisfies one's partner most, ask.

Obviously, intimate areas are sensitive and delicate, and too much pressure can be painful instead of pleasurable, especially for women. Men, on the other hand, can handle and often enjoy more pressure. Women require delicate touch and gentle squeezing of their vaginal areas, and the same goes for men's testicles, but an erect penis should be treated with more force. A good way to gauge what a partner likes is to observe his reactions, but an even better way is to communicate with each other and exchange information on what feels good and what to avoid. A careful explanation of each other's desires, reactions, and expectations, which can be done in a humorous way, can go a long way.

Many women get frustrated and avoid intimate massage, missing out on a healthy form of fun because they do not know much about it. As a result, their love lives become boring, and that should be a sign for change. Trying some new ideas in the bedroom may prove to be very refreshing, and it can awaken an appetite for sex. It is best to come up with one's own ideas, but it is okay to look for suggestions from outside sources. The purpose is to pleasure oneself and your partner. That way it is not a chore, but fun. And that is how it should be: intimate games; massage and sex should strengthen the relationship and make everyone happy. Many techniques may be important and useful but only if done with passion and closeness to each other.

Each person's mood is very important. The desire to pleasure one another, to play out each other's fantasies, and to try new things can bring great satisfaction. It is important to remember to engage in joyful bedroom antics devoid of any stress. Those playful moments should become an indispensable part of everyone's intimate lives. It is only normal to want to be creative in the bedroom. After all, we never cease to develop in many areas of our lives. So why should we in this particular one?

Intimate massage parlors offer many services, but they do not always live up to people's expectations. Many prefer to have a permanent masseuse who makes house calls. It does not matter where it is done; if it feels more comfortable at home than in a parlor, then by all means the important thing is for the masseuse to be a specialist in the type of massage performed. The presence of a professional is crucial because massage is not easy and can be done in many ways with the help of many accessories. A patient may have individual needs that a professional can properly address.

The services that we provide in our parlor are for both men and women—meaning a woman can come in for an erotic massage or she can be there to give one to a man. Couples are welcome too. For example, a man can get a massage and his woman can watch and learn, or she can perform the massage herself under the therapist's supervision. I have seen many women come in by themselves to learn the techniques of intimate massage.

There are many options, so everyone can draw joy from their intimacy. There is nothing wrong with wanting to satisfy one's erotic fantasies, as long as both people are consenting adults agreeing to be intimate with each other, and no one is forced to do anything.

What else can one expect from an intimate massage parlor? What further benefits can a person draw from seeing a professional masseuse? The answers to this and many other questions await in the following chapters.

CHAPTER 3

From Touch to Massage

The art of massage has a lot to do with learning a partner's "body map," which involves finding the most sensitive of the erogenous zones. These sensitive areas, as well as the order and method in which they should be stimulated must be explored through touching, caressing, massaging, observing a partner's reactions, and communicating with one another. Everybody has their own unique "body map," just like everyone has an original fingerprint. Because human beings are all different, with varying erogenous regions of the body, their reactions to outside stimuli are different as well. This explains why some women love to kiss and be kissed but caressing their breasts does not do much for them, while others love to have their bosoms touched, squeezed, licked, massaged, etc. This is why partners should take time to know each other and their intimate secrets, desires, and fantasies . . .

The maps of sensitive spots are similar for both sexes; however, their sensitivity is different. Women prefer neck, back, and arm massages while men are mostly content with intimate parts massages. When it comes to the art of massage, the learning process is crucial—and the theory has to be verified by practice, for individual preferences are more important than all the theoretical wisdom.

People are not always able to correctly read their partners' signals, in which case an honest conversation helps clear things up. By exchanging their observations (for instance, where to touch, how to touch), partners can quickly correct what they were doing wrong. By the way, that is a great exercise in openly talking about each other's intimate wants and needs. It is not as easy as it seems, even for many people in long-term relationships.

Sometimes one will have to make some changes when massaging because some assumptions will be different from the expectations of the partner. If that happens (and one should be ready for such a possibility), one has to immediately change something, such as the technique, the pressure, etc., so that it is to the partner's liking. A massage at home with a partner is much different than one done by a professional massage therapist, mainly because of the emotional bond present in the relationship. Knowledge and skills are not everything. Some initial awkwardness and minor mistakes are nothing next to such attributes as mutual closeness, or a feeling of safety, comfort, and trust. If two people come to understand their intimate adventures, they will find new meaning in them, and that is what matters.

The art of massage, whether relaxing, erotic, or intimate has the same basic rule: the more subtle the stimulus, the better the effect. An unforgettable sensory experience can be created through varying uses of brushing, petting, stroking, scratching, and other forms of touch. Sexual stimuli in the form of touching works for both partners—the one getting touched as well as the one touching. The best massage is one actively involving both people. Only then can the mutual efforts blossom into full pleasure.

To be able to experience such pleasure, the person getting the massage must trustfully give himself to the masseuse, who in turn tries to help him discover and fulfill his partner's expectations. While getting massaged one should be completely inactive, completely detached from the outside world, focused on and enjoying the pleasure of the massage. It is best to close one's eyes and concentrate on one's breathing, the massage, and the surrounding sounds. One should try not to think about anything. The only responsibility during the massage is to react to it, to let one's partner know what feels good and what doesn't. Always remember that patience is a virtue, and it might come in handy when learning the art of massage.

A person's mindset toward caressing plays an important role in the success. Even long-term stimulation of the most sensitive erogenous zones can be rendered ineffective with an indifferent— or even worse—or negative attitude.

When one learns massage needs and how to satisfy them, one will longingly await the next massage.

The touch

There are about a hundred thousand very-sensitive and more than half a million less-sensitive nerves in the human body. Nerve endings are located under the skin, but they connect all the organs in the body. A few hundred are unusually sensitive to outside stimuli such as touch and pressure.

The secret of touch is in the skin. It may seem hard to believe, but each person has natural healing powers in his or her touch. This is possible because of an inseparable bond between body and mind. This bond can be used in both directions—body to mind as well as mind to body—but that is a topic for a different book.

The strength of this book can be used to better someone's mood or health through relaxation.

Touch is a form of communication that does not require the use of words. It can be used to convey subtle information, such as feelings, optimism, or state of mood. It can have a comforting effect. The acceptation of touch is a meaningful proof of one's attitude toward another person.

Massage is a special kind of touch. It harnesses a positive energy, which has many benefits and helps solve many problems. For those close to one another it is a symbol of a bond and emotional involvement. Just like sex, it has a power to heal physically and emotionally. If it is targeted at a specific ailment it heals, and if it is used by a healthy individual it increases vital strength and betters the mood, acting as an excellent preventive treatment.

A physically arousing massage affects different bodily functions, such as breathing and circulation. It stimulates the respiratory gas exchange, which in turn can increase lung capacity. When taking in deep breaths, more oxygen reaches the lungs, from where it gets into the bloodstream. The genitals get a bigger than usual dose of blood, which causes arousal and an erection. The heart beats faster and blood rushes through the veins. The brain starts producing a range of chemical compounds (endorphins), which play a role in each person's well being. Endorphins act as a natural painkiller and strengthen the immune system. People whose bodies produce enough endorphins have fewer health problems, get sick less often, and generally feel better than those who have an endorphin deficiency. Thus, sensual touch, arousal, and sex can be great and enjoyable methods of feeling and being healthy. Experts on the subject claim that massage, or even sensuous touch, can have an effect similar to meditation or yoga.

One can derive pleasure from healing with massage and focus on improving other parts of their life. One should remember that emotions can spice up a sex life and affect one's mood. With the help of massage, a person can control or lesson the effects of migraines, asthma, a bad mood, skin problems, circulation problems, depression, and even chronic pain.

By taking time to learn massage, one is investing in the joy of life. An individual can feel this joy even though it is not tangible, but first one must get rid of things that stand in the way: stress, fear, tension, exhaustion, and others. Massage is supposed to take people to a different world. It has to be massage, not quick intercourse. The sex should wait until one learns to integrate it with massage to reach full satisfaction.

It turns out that the joy of intimate games improves women's self-confidence and helps them realize that the trivial things, which they considered priorities before, are not worth worrying about. Thanks to massage, things of little or no importance are no longer a source of distress. Instead, a stronger bond between two people can be established. The world does not change by itself, people do, and because of that they transform the world.

Those who persist in learning, and finally experience the change will always use intimate massage. And when a person starts feeling better because of it, then he can give in to his desires. Improved relations with a partner and the joy of giving and receiving pleasure can make one more enthusiastic and lively. When knowing how to give and receive, one can become a different person, and it also applies to the intimate part of life.

The so-called miracle recoveries most often take place in long-term, faithful relationships. Those relationships, based on honesty and trust, can be the source of healing powers in the intimate, as well as other areas of life. Physical illness can be influenced not only through physical means. The satisfaction from one's love life restores the joy of life and betters the health. This book is not only a tutorial of intimate massage, it also puts an emphasis on showing the importance of a strong bond and its effects on the process of healing.

Intimate games create a perfect opportunity to experience the healing power of touch. For many, especially men, sexual contact is the only chance to freely touch and be touched, but keep in mind that even a simple hug brings nothing but benefits.

<u>Side note</u>

Touch plays a crucial role in each life. What happens when a man is touched by a virgin? Ancient tradition sheds some light on this matter. People in antiquity used to believe in the unusual power of virgins. Many accounts from the old days tell of tales about virgin temples and legendary vestal virgins. They were considered personifications of godly powers because they were able to restrain from sex. Even in our times a virgin is considered a symbol of purity.

In the ancient accounts, the virgins participated in a practice called shunamitism (the name is derived from the biblical town of Shunam). This practice is based on the belief in sexual energy. This is an extraordinary energy that a man can receive through close contact with a virgin. This energy is transferred by lying naked next to each other. Sex is forbidden in this practice because it would nullify the specific energy flow.

There are many examples of shunamitism(7). According to the followers of this practice, a Roman citizen by the name of Claudius

Hermippus lived to be 115 years old because he slept with virgins but did not have sex with them.

A certain eighteenth-century house of shunamitism in Paris was very popular. Madame Janus, the host, employed more than fifty virgins who took care of their clients in various ways, excluding sex. If a client tried to convince the girls to have intercourse with him, he would be heavily fined. Men could enjoy the services provided by the girls, which included bathing, rubbing on fragrant oils, and massaging. Finally, they would lead him to bed, where he would lie between them.

A variety of shunamitism are the so-called Brahmacharya experiments practiced in India and other countries of the region. The purpose of this practice is to sleep in the company of naked girls for warmth. The best-known supporter and practitioner of Brahmacharya was Gandhi**(8)**.

Mentions of shunamitism are found in the Old Testament, and that's probably how the practice started and spread around the world. Here is an excerpt from the scriptures describing the situation that gave birth to this practice:

King David was old and stricken in years; and they covered him with clothes, but he got no heat. Let there be sought for my Lord the king a young virgin: and let her stand before the king, and let her cherish him, and let her lie in thy bosom, that my lord the king may get heat. So they sought for a fair damsel throughout all the coasts of Israel, and found Abishag a Shunamite, and brought her to the king. And the damsel was very fair, and cherished the king, and ministered to him: but the king knew her not.—
1 Book of Kings 1:1-4

The healing touch

The healing touch is called a caress, and it is a delicate touch, different from massaging and squeezing. Certain conditions must be met in order for healing to take place:

- It has to be done very slowly, about half as fast as normal.
- It cannot cause tension.
- It requires concentration on the task at hand. It is important to be aware of the present and to not drift in thought. This is not easy, especially during longer sessions. If one catches himself thinking about the past or the future during a session, he should try to switch to thinking about his current feelings.
- It has to be pleasurable.

There are many massage techniques, but they are all based on the use of systematic movements. These movements are rubbing, petting, squeezing, and tapping of the skin. Massage can be combined with other therapies, such as aromatherapy, hydrotherapy, and so on.

A simple massage can be performed by almost anybody.

What are the benefits of massage?

Massage can:

- Bring more blood, and in consequence more oxygen and nutrients to the tissue, improving its quality.
- Improve circulation, which prevents the creation of varicose veins.

- Remove byproducts of metabolism and the toxins gathered in stiff muscles.
- Improve the agility of muscles.
- Decrease muscle aches by stretching and relaxing the muscles.
- Stimulate the lymphatic system.
- Improve the skin, increasing blood flow to it, remove callous skin.
- Remove excess water from intercellular areas.
- Help heal scars.*
- Soothe the nerves.
- Add vitality.
- Eliminate stress and fatigue.
- Regulate blood pressure.
- Decrease or eliminate headaches, backaches, and pains in the spine.
- Bring about a good mood.
- Ease a variety of pains.
- Decrease stress that accumulates throughout the day.
- Strengthen the immune system if performed on a regular basis.
- Help the natural flow of energy in the body, eliminating phantom pains.

Time for massage

It is best to start with a sensuous massage. It does not matter what position one starts in. One can lie down next to his partner and caress each other; however, one person must eventually take up the initiative to start the actual massage, where one person becomes the giver and the other the receiver. If the goal of the massage is just pleasure, then the course of action is totally up to the partners, but if the purpose is something else, discipline is a must. For example, heightened arousal cannot be a reason to stop the massage and seek satisfaction. A massage is like a feast for both body and spirit, but certain preparations must be made. A person should put much effort into the massage preparation, just as one would when cooking a meal, and when all is ready one can indulge in the feast.

Preparing the area

Not much space is needed for a massage; a bed or bedroom floor are usually fine. A massage can be done outdoors provided it is warm enough and there is privacy. The latter is important, especially if one lives with other people. Most of the time living with other people in the same house does not pose a problem since intimate games usually take place at night. There is a certain downside to bedroom adventures at night. People may be tired by then. When choosing a place for the massage, remember to have enough room for the masseuse to be comfortable too. It is not good if one cannot concentrate on massaging because of discomfort.

Lighting

Massage has to be performed in a casual atmosphere, so dim lighting is preferred. There should be just enough light to see what one is doing, so complete darkness is not recommended. Seeing each other naked and excited stimulates the senses. Candlelight is soothing and romantic, and can definitely be used.

Most of the masseurs from the east were blind, and because of their handicap they had a highly developed sense of touch. If someone feels uncomfortable being naked in the light, one has to work on it in little steps because it may not always be possible to massage or make love at night. To eliminate the discomfort, one should start out with very little light that he can accept. With each massage, one turns it up a little until reaching a level of lighting optimal for both partners. Remember that bright light has a tendency to distract, while dim lighting has a romantic effect.

Setting the mood

It helps to have some things handy that can help get in the mood when preparing for a massage. Having scented candles, incense, or multiple fragrant oils within reach, or anything else that works is a good idea. Appropriate music might be a big help. There are many romantic or relaxing compilations out there that are perfect for intimate moments. Some people prefer instrumental music. Having a TV on during a massage is not a good idea because the combination of picture and sound can distract. Radio is also not recommended, since music is often interrupted with commentary, conversations, and commercials, which is also distracting and possibly frustrating.

It is definitely a plus to have a fireplace in the house. It provides warmth, light, and a unique mood. Just like candlelight, it creates a romantic setting.

Additional accessories

Before starting a massage, a person will need to get some essential things ready: towels, bathrobes, balms and oils, and if desired, some wine. One can also use a wide variety of accessories, such as feathers, brushes, pieces of fur or silk, a vibrator, etc. Massage therapy can also be enriched with aromatherapeutic oils, balsams, or talcum powder. Many of those things are used to make the contact between the hands and the body smoother and more enjoyable. One does not have to use a lot of lubricant, just enough to spread over the body or the area to be massaged. It is good if the oil is slightly warm. As a rule one should not pour oils directly on to the partner's skin, but it all depends on the situation. Sometimes pouring a lubricant from an appropriate height onto the body might be intriguing. When aroused, a small stream of oil spilled on the frenulum or the clitoris as well as the nipples can be very pleasurable.

Sharing a bath

It is an important element of massage, contributing to the good mood of both partners. A mutual fragrant bath by candlelight and quiet music can set the mood for the massage and the rest of the evening. Using a loofah, sponge, brush, or a terrycloth mitten on each other during the bath can be an excellent introduction to a sensual, intimate, or erotic massage. After the bath, dry each other off and proceed to the massaging station. Remember to remove all jewelry before the bath but definitely before the massage.

Using the hair

If either partner has long hair one can use it to pleasure the other by running its tips along their body. It is a great way to turn the heat up a little, especially if one uses it on the inner side of arms and legs. Of course it also works great on other body parts, such as the back and torso.

The basic massage tools are the hands. They have to be smooth and delicate, and the nails should be short and rounded so they do not hurt one's partner. It is true that long nails, if properly used, can be a source of pleasure. Light scratching or dragging them across the skin, especially with the outer side of the hand, is definitely worth a try.

Delicate movements

These movements are used most often in intimate massages. They are easy to learn because all one does is barely touch the surface of the partner's skin as one slowly moves the hands along it. Delicate movements are ideal for the beginning and the end of the massage. Use them along the whole body and do not concentrate on one spot. These moves should be very gentle in order to produce a calming effect. The use of massage oil is encouraged. Instead of using the whole hand, try just the fingertips, but be careful not to do it too lightly, as it may start to tickle and spoil the moment. Experiment with each other and see what feels good. Use both hands or alternate fingertips, move them along the body, or make circles and other shapes—the possibilities are endless.

Sliding movements

These types of moves are undoubtedly pleasing. While standing at the partner's feet or head, one slides the hands with palms flat as far down his or her partner's body as possible and then slides them back. This way different body parts are affected simultaneously.

Another version of a sliding movement is to use one's palms in a circular motion. A person can alternate hands, using one for bigger circles and the other for smaller, with a common center point.

One should remember to always keep one hand in contact with the partner's body, not just when using sliding moves but throughout the entire massage. After learning these exercises and their basic rules, one can and most definitely will be able to explore one's own ideas and create unique versions. The key to lots of fun here is to use the imagination and be inventive.

Side note

Although there are many techniques, schools, and different philosophies regarding massage, one thing has been proven: touch, as long as it is performed with love, no matter the style of massage, is good for the health. One of the scientists from the University of Ohio(9) performed the following experiment: he fed two groups of rabbits food rich in cholesterol, but only some were pet and caressed. As a result, the rabbits that were touched had a 50 percent less probability of developing arteriosclerosis than those that were kept devoid of touch.

CHAPTER 4

Similarities in the Erogenous Zones

Certain parts of the human body are especially sensitive to touch. Even though men and women have different sexual reactions, both sexes share the same sensitive areas on their bodies. Men who think the only source of pleasure on their bodies is their reproductive organ are really missing out.

Starting from the top, the first erogenous zone is the ears, so remember to gently play with them. Next on the list are the lips, a symbol of kissing, and an obvious epicenter of pleasure. The nape of the neck and inner arms are sensitive to touch. Stimulating the chest, including the breasts and nipples, is exciting too, and not just for women! The lower abdomen is another place to touch if one wants to arouse a partner. When it comes to the buttocks, a firmer form of stimulation is usually preferred. Inner thighs and the back of the knees are good places to touch as well. A foot massage, with the focus on the big toe, can be very enjoyable.

Just because those areas are more sensitive than others does not mean one should concentrate only on them. But when a person does touch them, it should not be done just to get a sexual reaction. The touch is supposed to be a way to communicate, a language between two people, symbolizing a strong bond and a feeling of safety.

Erogenous zones are important areas of the body for all, especially in intimate lives, but also during massages. The purpose of "therapy" by intimate massage is to maintain arousal for a specific period of time through the stimulation of erogenous zones. Knowing those zones and not just the ones deemed most important is priceless, because if during a massage a patient gets too aroused it is better to switch to a less sensitive area than to pause the massage. This rule applies to almost all situations, with only a few exceptions. For instance, if a man is too excited or he is extremely sensitive to touch.

The course of a massage will be different with each session, depending on the relationship of the people; for example, a kiss during a session will not be acceptable unless the persons involved are emotionally close to each other. Such behavior in a professional setting is unacceptable.

It is commonly believed that men have fewer erogenous zones than women. This incorrect opinion is an effect of a misunderstanding caused by the differences in sensitivity of the erogenous zones between the two sexes. It would be wrong to assume that the stimulation of a woman's breasts will have the same effect as the stimulation of a man's chest. Usually breasts are more sensitive to caressing, but men can also enjoy a chest massage.

Just touching the erogenous zones is an attractive form of massage. Touching and caressing should be done with slight and delicate movements. Long strokes have a soothing, calming effect. Such a massage affects a person's mood, is relaxing, and finally, it can stimulate sexually. Delicate petting, as well as stimulating caressing, can be an introduction to a massage or an intoxicating night. This subtle contact can encourage disclosing deepest desires and sexual fantasies. It allows opening up to a partner, creates more trust, and strengthens the relationship.

First, let's go over men's erogenous zones—because women's sensitivity is a bit more complicated. Understanding men's erogenous zones will make it easier to understand how they work in women.

The ears

This body part is absolutely unappreciated by women. Many men feel that ear stimulation is a sign of affection toward a partner. Touching the ears with the fingers or tongue is most effective when done with passion. Some men like to have their inner part of the ears sucked or licked.

The face

A warm breath or a brush of the tongue on the face can stimulate the senses and arouse a partner. Gently caressing a partner's face with the hands and tapping it with the fingers relaxes and stimulates the muscles. A method born in India called butterfly kisses is a fun and exciting "massage," which is performed by tickling a partner's lips, nose, and the nape of the neck with the eyelashes.

The nape of the neck

This area is very sensitive to touch, especially at the hairline. Men enjoy having the area between the hairline and the shoulders kissed and caressed. Gentle biting in this area is an arousing experience.

In order to arouse and make a man enjoy a massage, his partner has to locate and skillfully stimulate the erogenous zones. To make the experience enjoyable, it is necessary to pet, kiss, and tickle the chest, lips, and other sensitive spots with the tip of the tongue. Brushing the hands along the skin, digging the nails into the skin, and biting also arouses many men.

Especially sensitive areas on a man's body are the nipples, the front of the shoulders, and upper and mid back. Just like women, men have other sensitive areas aside from the genitals. These spots are located all along the body, from the lips, ears, and the neck especially near the hairline, to the hands, butt, and feet.

The nipples

Men's nipples are not as sensitive as women's—same goes for the whole chest—but they are receptive to touch and can be a source of interesting sensations. Some men like to have their nipples pulled and twisted. A proper way of stimulating the lower back and buttocks areas may lead a man to increased arousal. It is especially exciting for a man to have those areas of his body kissed and licked by his partner while she is simultaneously stimulating his penis.

Another erogenous zone on a man's body stretches from the armpits down to the hips. Using the fingertips, lips, hands, and tongue to gently touch this area can generate a very nice sensation. Moving this stimulation toward the member will increase a man's arousal.

The spine

The skin along the spine is also sensitive to touch, and if stimulated correctly it can have very desirable effects. Use the fingertips or nails to barely touch the skin along the spine as one move, from the neck to the butt; very exciting.

Inner thighs

The most sensitive area on the inner thigh stretches from the middle of the thigh to the crotch. Caressing or tickling this area causes quick arousal. Stimulation performed in this area with the tongue and lips, especially near the penis, is very exciting. The crotch, a very sensitive spot, is located between the anal sphincter and the base of the scrotum.

The sex organs

The skin of the scrotum has many nerve endings, which is why a man is quick to react to its caressing. Such touching can be gentle or firm—what is important is that it should not cause pain. The type of massage used depends on both people involved. For example, a woman may choose movements ranging from a skim of a finger to a stroke of a hand while simultaneously alternating gentle and firm squeezing of the genitals. A man may enjoy the stretching of the scrotum combined with retracting the foreskin and moving the testicles up and down. As one can see, there is a wide range of types of touch to choose from. One can also alternate the different types of stimulation: by awakening a man's senses in one area of his body and then switching to another, only to come back to the previous one.

The places that are especially sensitive to touch are the ones that have many nerve endings running through them, perhaps partially innervating them. Sensitive to the touch is also the area surrounding the anus and the skin along the penile raphe (a visible line or ridge of tissue that extends from the anus to the perineum). Stroking and teasing this area with the fingers creates intense sensations and causes a violent flow of blood to the lymphatic vessels of the penis.

The penis is right next to the testes, and its stimulation can take on different forms. If the member is soft and one wants to get it hard and rigid quickly, a person can apply gentle pressure with the whole hand and massage the penis from the base up. The back side of the penis is very sensitive to touch, especially where the scrotal raphe runs from the crotch and the scrotum. This raphe culminates at the frenulum of prepuce, which is a fold of skin that fixes the foreskin to the tip of the member. These areas are the most sensitive.

Tickling, touching, and caressing the intimate erogenous zones excites any man. Such caressing has two purposes: it causes the man some pleasure while at the same time exciting the woman, who experiences the swelling, rising, and hardening of the penis caused by her massage. These experiences are very arousing, especially for women who are already experienced in lovemaking. The hardening of the member and its erection are tangible proof of the sexual impingement a woman has on a man, and there is no greater disaster in the emotional-erotic life of a woman than a situation during which the man stops positively reacting to her caressing.

The ladies and their erogenous zones

The lips

The first erogenous area that partners usually explore together is the lips. This experience brings them back to their early childhood, when many pleasant sensations are experienced through that part of the body. Babies love to come into contact not only with their mothers' breasts but with other things, such as food, their own fingers, and toys, sheets, and any other objects they first put in their mouth, because for them it is the best way of familiarizing themselves with those objects.

The face

Next we explore the face. The area around the nostrils is as sensitive as the lips. The skin between the nose and the upper lip, as well as the skin between the lower lip and the chin is usually covered with more peach fuzz than other areas of the body and as a result of gently touching those places, the tiny hairs stand up and the person feels aroused.

The head

The areas of the head, neck, and ears—stroking those places causes very pleasant sensations in most women. A man's hand moving across a woman's nape of the neck is a very pleasurable and arousing experience. Playing with a partner's hair is also quite attractive. Skimming the nape of the neck with the tongue, or breathing warm air on that body part releases a partner's reactions. Therefore, a massage—regardless of the type—should be started from the head and neck. The delicate caressing of the nape of the neck and the neck itself intensify arousal, whet the sexual appetite, and stimulate a woman to erotic activities and games. Touching, stroking, and caressing those places causes feelings of sensual pleasure.

The breasts

The path of caressing through the neck, the nape of the neck, shoulders, back, and armpits leads to the breasts. There are two very important spots above and below the bosom, equipped with special receptors. Skillfully applying pressure to these points with the fingertips causes increased hormonal production in a woman's body. A woman's breasts are not only essential attributes of her beauty and are not only a guarantee of health and proper development of her future children, they are also her richest, most subtle, and sensitive instrument of erotic emotion. The breasts, like the most sensitive photocell, react to even a trace of heat, touch, or other love signals. The bosom of women that is not aroused droops just a little bit, but just a thought about her lover, his glance at her, or perhaps brushing against his body initiates the erotic game on the cellular level, causing increased blood flow, and therefore, the raising and filling out of the breasts. Breasts filled out and tensed with blood are more sensitive to caressing and touching.

Grabbing a breast with the whole hand excites a man as well as a woman when the palm of his hand brushes against her nipple. Caressing the breasts should be gentle—first with the fingertips, using circular movements from the outside of the breasts, in toward the nipple. Gentle biting, kissing, and sucking create unforgettable moments. Nipples can be stimulated in many different ways—from licking and tickling, to gentle pinching and biting. Light and interrupted skimming of the nipples with the whole hand, the fingertips, or rubbing the nipples against the naked skin of a man causes them to "stand up." This happens because the elastic fibers in the connective tissue around the areolas and nipples shrink, causing the areolas to get smaller and the nipples to harden and protrude.

There is a kind of breast stimulation that brings a lot of satisfaction to both partners. The nipples get tickled and caressed with the tip of an erect penis. The tactile stimuli in this kind of caressing are very arousing. It is, however, quite a refined massage technique, most appropriate for mature and experienced relationships.

When it comes to breast stimulation there is one rule: the more gentle and subtle the stimulus, the better the effect, and the stronger the sensation. Breast massage brings most women positive experiences and much pleasure, provided her partner is not pesky about it or does not manifest brutality in the stimulation. This is because women are much more sensitive to touch than men. Caressing that is brutal or too strong hurts and discourages instead of being arousing. The exceptions to that rule are obese women whose nerve endings are isolated by a layer of fat. In those cases, harder spanking and pinching can have similar positive effects to the delicate caressing of most women.

An aroused man oftentimes displays a tendency to painfully squeezing or biting a woman's breasts. Therefore, remember that this technique of massage does not always bring the desired results and that aroused and thus swollen breasts are very sensitive and prone to injury. If a massage is performed in a manner that is too powerful, the effect is painful and the woman is usually discouraged from continuing. The best advice for men in such a case is to calm down, relax, and follow his intuition. A massage should begin with gentle touching, and only after some time somewhat stronger stimuli can be used—when the woman gets used to the arousal and the contact with the man's hand.

The spine

The outer sides of the arms right above the elbows have two spots, which react to temperature changes and have a calming affect on the overall mood just by touching them with warm hands and applying a little bit of gentle pressure. The loins on either side of the spine contain two important spots that are often used in acupuncture. Massaging those spots regenerates weakened strength and vitality. Another two spots are located about an inch above the tailbone. When stimulated, they tend to cause sexual readiness in a woman.

The abdomen

If a partner is tense, spend a little more time on a relaxing caress of the abdomen and waist, especially around the navel. Applying gentle pressure in that area calms and relaxes, causing strong reactions. The touch of warm hands along the sides of the torso, as well as brushing of the tongue and playing with a warm breath in those spots brings extraordinary results. Those methods make the skin react and cause a thrill for a partner.

The intimate areas

The wandering hand should be directed toward the intimate area, along the vulva, where it encounters the labia minora and the clitoris. By tickling and caressing it, the clit will become perceptible as an elongated, hard "roller" with the thickness of about one small finger.

It is worth to remember that women, generally, prefer gentle, steady stimulation. But sometimes a continuous, uniform motion causes a decrease of arousal. In this case, a man should switch to a different type of stimulus. When massaging a partner's intimate areas, remember to vary the type of stimulation.

Tickling the clitoris can cause an orgasm by teaching a partner how to enjoy the experience even long before the first intercourse; therefore, this massage is recommended for girls who are still afraid to start having sex. Such experiences decrease the fear of the "first time" and awaken the curiosity of other erotic acts.

The buttocks

An acupressure massage of the buttocks can be very rewarding because it simultaneously relaxes and arouses. Such a massage should be gentle but firm. Tender stretching of the skin, light pinching, or making circles with the fingertips on both buttocks enables a woman to calm down and relax, causing her to completely trust her masseur.

The thighs

The inner thighs of a woman are characterized by exceptional sensitivity. In some women an orgasm can be caused just by kissing and caressing the thighs and the knees. Those areas contain spots where applying pressure helps decrease menstrual cramps. The use of these spots can do wonders and cause genuine gratitude and admiration from one's partner.

There is a magical spot that increases the sexual drive. It is located in the middle of the leg, right below and behind the kneecap.

Applying delicate pressure to this spot can revive even the most tired lover.

There are countless possibilities when it comes to caressing different body parts. One can brush them tenderly, caress them with one's mouth, and gently blow air on them. The important thing is that what someone does should bring pleasure to the person being touched. Turn on the imagination and think up new ways of showing a partner the devotion and feelings. When a person touches a loved one, he makes her happy. Partners channel a feeling of well being, affection, and give satisfaction and relaxation.

A man should try to make a sexual portrait of his lover in his head, kind of like a map of the different erogenous zones and other important areas of her body. When caressing her hands, face, shoulders, and ears one should try to maximize the effects by slowing down and really focusing on those areas. The reactivity of each of the receptors must be awakened through diligent massage so that they clearly respond to caressing. Obvious excitability is rarely found in this area, especially in young women. Learning to caress and be caressed develops a hidden sensitivity to touch. For example, a woman who, after many years of boring intercourse with a primitive and selfish man, blossoms under the friendly hand of a gentle partner.

The Kegel muscle

A sedentary lifestyle that has become the norm for many of us leaves our physical fitness with much to be desired. It is not just our physical dexterity that suffers, but our lack of sexual prowess has become an Achilles' heel for many. Of course going to the gym can exercise many of the muscles and improve our physical appearance, but the key to improving the quality of our intimate lives is a muscle many people cannot even find. It is the *pubococcygeus muscle*, also called the PC muscle, but most commonly known as the Kegel muscle. The name of this muscle comes from a doctor by the name of Arnold Kegel who, in the 1940s, compiled a special set of exercises for women suffering from bladder malfunction. These exercises were designed to control the excretion of urine through the contraction of proper muscles. It then became apparent that the strengthening of those muscles not only prevents the leakage of urine but eases childbirth and increases sexual pleasure in both sexes. It is about time to intensify the sensations!

In order to exercise the Kegel muscle, one must locate it first. The easiest way to do it is to place the fingers on the labium* and try to hold back urine. The muscle that is squeezed during the process is the Kegel. When contracting, it is important to relax the muscles of the thighs and abdomen and to breathe calmly. This exercise, as opposed to working out at the gym, should be practically unnoticeable on the outside.

Examples of basic exercises

1. Contract and relax the PC muscle twenty times. It is a good idea to repeat this exercise three times a day. The advantage of this exercise is that it can be done during normal, everyday circumstances, such as waiting in line, brushing your teeth, watching TV, etc.
2. Squeeze the Kegel muscle, hold it for three seconds, and relax it. Repeat ten times.
3. Contract the Kegel muscle as you take a breath. While doing so, focus on trying not to squeeze your abdominal muscles, which can pose a problem at first—but it is just a matter of practice before you master it.

If you do these exercises regularly you will quickly notice results. The vaginal opening will have better "tension" and will increase your pleasure, even if your partner is not very large. As a result of these exercises, your partner will also experience more intense sensations. Squeezing the penis with your Kegel after an ejaculation can even let your man maintain an erection, allowing another go at it after a quick rest, without taking the member out of the vagina. Of course in order to attain such results, you have to conduct these exercises for several months.

Advanced exercises

1. **Moving your hips.** Stand with your legs slightly apart, your hands on your hips, and make circular movements (as large as you can) with your hips, first to the left, and then in the opposite direction. Do this very smoothly and repeat about twenty to thirty sets. This exercise helps relax the hips and therefore to better receive sexual stimuli.

2. **Pushing out the hips.** Push your hips out in both directions, first to the front, and then to the back with your abdominal and leg muscles completely relaxed. This exercise can be performed while standing up or lying down.

3. **Hip thrusts.** When lying down, bring up your knees and thrust your hips up and down. Since your whole back is pressed along the surface you're lying on, your freedom of movement is limited. In the "standing" version of this exercise make sure your back remains motionless.

The Kegel in men

Let's start with locating the Kegel muscle before proceeding to the description of its role and significance for sexual prowess. To find the location of this muscle, place two fingers right behind the testicles and imagine that you are trying to stop a stream of urine. The muscle that you feel contracting at that moment is the Kegel. Repeat this "experiment" a few more times so you will not have any trouble locating it in the future. Now that you know where to find this muscle, you are probably wondering about its significance. Well, it helps to control premature ejaculations, make the ejaculation more plentiful, and allows the erection to be harder and last longer. The genitals become more sensitive to touch, orgasms intensify, and one might even be able to have multiple orgasms. Looking at this from a health perspective, the good form of the Kegel muscle contributes to maintaining the good health of the prostate, preventing it from enlarging.

Basic exercises

You should not get discouraged with the fact that at first you have little control over this muscle—because regular exercises will change that.

1. Concentrate and do ten to twenty repetitions of the Kegel muscle contraction. If the muscle tires quickly, it means it is out of shape and the only way to change that is consistency.
2. Squeeze the muscle as hard as you can and hold it for as long as possible.
3. Contract and relax your sphincter thirty times. Take a break for thirty seconds and then repeat the process twice more.

Try to get so good at this that you will be able to do a hundred or more repetitions in one set. The Kegel muscle quickly gets used to physical effort, so three hundred contractions a day should become the norm, guaranteeing you top sexual form well into your senior years.

For advanced users

This exercise, repeated regularly, will allow you to have "steely" and long-lasting erections.

Start with a warm up in the form of about thirty contractions of the Kegel muscle. Next, squeeze it once as hard as you can and hold it for twenty seconds. Then take a thirty second break and repeat this five times. After persistent training, you will be able to hold the muscle contracted even for a few minutes!

Exercise: the Kegel muscle in the role of sexual self-discipline

If you persistently exercise the Kegel muscle, it will become your ally when one-on-one with your partner. It will allow you to restrain a quickly growing arousal and therefore let you and your partner enjoy the pleasure that comes from it for a longer period of time. Choose a method of squeezing that suits you the most and use it every time you need it.

- One strong and one long squeeze
- Two medium contractions
- A few quick contractions, similar to those during an ejaculation

While squeezing the Kegel, try not to lose the erection. It is the best to master the chosen technique alone at first and, when you feel ready to try it out with your partner, ask her to start caressing you. Then she should massage you orally until you reach a high level of arousal. Then, squeeze the Kegel muscle until you go down a level on the arousal scale, relax the muscle, and let your partner continue the stimulation. When you feel that you have mastered this method, try to restrain your arousal right before the anticipated ejaculation.

Now you can consider yourself to have full control over your arousal. If that is really the case—just like in any situation where power is involved—do not abuse it. Sometimes just let it go and do not use your newly acquired ability to steer your sexual energy when with your partner, because abusing it can lead to temporary problems with your erection.

CHAPTER 5

It Is Worth Knowing . . .

How does a man's sexual reaction process compare to a woman's? The two models, first described in 1966 by a pair of sexologists by the names of William Masters and Virginia Johnson, are similar to each other. According to their theory, there are four stages of sexual response: arousal, plateau, orgasm, and relaxation.

In men, the first stage is accompanied by an erection, caused by a blood surge to the penis. After that, provided the outside stimuli are not stopped and the erection is kept up, the second stage, the plateau, starts. During this phase the erection becomes hard and the color of the penis intensifies. A few drops of pre-cum, which is not to be confused with semen, may appear. The third stage is an orgasm. When it is reached, the Kegel and pelvis muscles cramp up. Just like during a female orgasm, blood pressure violently increases, as do the heartbeat and breathing rate. These reactions suddenly subside at the culmination point. In most cases, an orgasm is accompanied by an ejaculation and followed by a fading of the erection. The body becomes desensitized to sexual stimuli for a period of time that varies from a few minutes to a few hours. Although a climax and an ejaculation usually occur together, it is possible to have an orgasm without an ejaculation. It is called a dry orgasm. Such an occurrence can take place if a man climaxes a few times in a short span of time, as a result of taking certain prescription medications or illicit drugs, or because of a young age, when there is no semen to be produced yet.

Both sexes experience the same stages of the sexual cycle, but the main difference between the two is the time it takes to reach an orgasm. Very few women are capable of climaxing almost right away. When it comes to men, that attribute is a lot more common, especially when it comes to young individuals who have not yet learned to control their sexual reactions. The famous *Dr. Kinsey Reports* state that it takes as little as ten seconds for some individuals to have an orgasm. The inability to hold back an ejaculation may lead to thoughts of the impossibility of satisfying a partner, which, in turn, might lead to serious insecurities.

When it comes to multiple orgasms, another dissonance appears. Even though a woman can have multiple orgasms during the same intercourse, such an occurrence is rare in men.

It may come as a surprise, but faking an orgasm is not just a female "skill." One may ask, "How is that? It is possible to fake an ejaculation?" Of course not, but an aroused woman's vagina produces enough moisture for a lack of sperm to remain unnoticed with the use of some acting skills. But why would a man want to fake an orgasm? Well, perhaps during sex a man starts to feel that he is losing his erection and does not want to "compromise his manhood." In order to save face and avoid embarrassment, he fakes it.

A little bit of anatomy

Usually for men, the most important body part is their penis. They think that without it, they would stop being a source of interest for women. That is why men pamper their best friend so much.

The term "penis" comes from the Latin word for "tail." A flaccid member usually varies in size from 3.3 to 4.1 inches, with an average of 3.7 inches. An erect penis grows on average 2.9 inches, which makes an average erection 4.9 to 6.9 inches, with a circumference of 3.7 inches. As a rule, a small, flaccid member grows more in length, percentage-wise, in comparison to a large one also starting in a state of rest.

During an ejaculation a man usually excretes about a teaspoonful of semen. The amount of sperm given off during an orgasm can vary—depending on the frequency of intercourse, the state of health, as well as many other factors. Women should not think they can tell if a man is being faithful based on the amount of sperm ejaculated.

An important warning to women. If a woman wants to have a man's respect and affection, she should never allow herself any mockery about his limp penis. When it is erect and hard she can talk and laugh about it, but never when it is soft and flaccid. Many men are sensitive about this issue, and this is why many turn their backs to their partners after intercourse. They are just not impressed with the appearance of their member and do not want their partner to see a "small, helpless sausage."

When on the move, a man's member is placed not straight but to one side. Most men "hang" to the left; so, if one would like to massage it through the clothing, it is best to keep that in mind. It is within reach of an arm when standing in front of the partner. Never bend an erect penis without checking with your partner and do not use any positions that may accidentally cause bending, unless you are sure it is fine to do so, as it may cause some unpleasant consequences.

If one has a cold sore on a lip, any oral sex should be avoided until it is gone because it can be transferred to the genitals, where it is harder to heal.

The tip of a penis has the most sensitive nerve endings—that is why a woman performing oral sex should pay close attention to that area licking and gently sucking it. Most men in the United States are circumcised and their tips are constantly exposed, but in recent years parents who are not motivated by tradition decide to leave their sons' penises intact. The foreskin just retracts during an erection. There is no difference in sensitivity between a circumcised and an uncircumcised man, although some people claim otherwise.

Men love it when women touch, hold, and squeeze their penises. It is a source of pleasure and satisfaction. Thus, even an accidental touch does not go unnoticed. It does not mean that there is an instantaneous erection, but thoughts start focusing on sex. An accidental touch does not necessarily have to be that accidental though.

The testicles are one of the most sensitive parts of a man's body. Their function has a great impact on sexuality, fertility, and mood. Usually the left testicle hangs a bit lower than the right. The opposite is usually true for left-handed men. When aroused, the testes increase in size usually by about 50 percent.

The scrotum has many sensitive nerve endings, so a man reacts quickly to its stimulation. The petting of the sack can be gentle and firm, but it is important that it does not hurt. Stretching the sack is a very pleasurable experience and at the same time it retracts the foreskin (if present). When a man is lying on his back, pulling the sack causes the penis to rise to an upright position. When the sack is released, the member "lies down." Such games can be as arousing for a man as for a woman. "Juggling" the balls and raising and lowering them causes pleasure for both partners too.

It is astonishing that so many women ignore the testicles in intimate play. Usually it is because they are afraid of hurting them—and that fear is not unjustified. Even the toughest man will tear up if his balls are squeezed too hard, but it does not mean a woman should not touch them. She should do it but skillfully. It is especially encouraged during an oral massage. Such a massage combined with stimulation of the testicles is a pleasure no man could easily forget. The sack can also be stimulated with the mouth, with licking and gentle sucking.

Men and women are baffled when they find out men also have a G-spot. Its exact location is hard to describe. It is a point located between the back of the scrotum and the anus. When moving a finger along that area look for a small indent and press it. One should feel a small bump; that is the G-spot on a man. The G-spot is one of the erogenous zones, which can be used in an intimate massage. But it is not only an erogenous zone; it also serves another purpose. It delays an erection and ejaculation if necessary. That and many other methods have been described in the section of the book pertaining to the subject (see Chapter 12 for more information).

The difference between sperm and pre-ejaculation fluid (pre-cum)

The production of sperm requires a colder setting than normal body temperature, and that is why the scrotum is wrinkled. It cools down the testes while retaining the heat in the sack itself. The scrotum stays warm while the testicles shrink because of the cooler temperature.

After the sperm is created in the testicles, it travels through a canal where it is mixed with the pre-ejaculatory fluid, which comes from the prostate. Pre-ejaculation fluid is very important because it serves as food and protection for the sperm, keeping it alive for the journey ahead. When the member is sufficiently aroused, the liquid travels through its center, causing a reaction in certain muscles. Finally the seed is thrown out in several spurts, up to a distance of five feet.

During an erection, the canal connecting the penis with the bladder contracts so that no urine gets through during sex.

Orgasm

The scale of men's sensations can be as rich as that of women's—from the typical satisfaction to an ecstasy of delight. Men react faster to sexual stimuli and do not need as much foreplay as women. It does not mean they do not need it at all. If a man does not suffer from any sexual disorders, he always has an ejaculation and therefore is relaxed, but it is hard to tell if he is fully satisfied.

Men, like women, experience better orgasms with a trusted partner they care about than a complete stranger. A casual adventure is a way to unload some sexual tension. A man experiences the most pleasure when he loves the woman he is with, he is happy with her, and when she is affectionate, accepting, and understanding toward him. Love in men, not unlike in women, can mature over a lifetime and only after many years of experience can reach its full capacity in the bedroom.

An ejaculation-free orgasm

Men can enjoy sex even without ejaculating. Eastern love technique specialists even encourage limiting ejaculations, claiming vital powers are freed along with the seed. TAO* masters formulated different rules of ejaculation frequencies. They claimed that a twenty-year old man can attain good health and longevity by limiting himself to two ejaculations a month, twenty-four a year. In addition to that, if he eats healthy and exercises, he is sure to live a long time.

Specialists also claim that men should limit how often they ejaculate after reaching the age of forty or fifty. Such restraint will guarantee the power and energy to increase the frequency and length of intercourse. This will allow both partners to feel more joy from sex, experience more devotion to each other, and be healthier and more relaxed. They will simply attain harmony in relations with each other.

Side note

Men, like women, are affected by many factors that decide their interest or aversion to bedroom issues. Professional, home, or financial problems often affect that area of life.

It is a known fact that certain types of work have a negative effect on love lives. However, nobody conducted any studies to find out which jobs affect human libido the most. In recent years those studies have been performed and the results show that men working in the financial and business sectors, as well as lawyers and doctors, are most prone to sexual problems. Politicians are also at risk.

Farming seems to be the most favorable profession when it comes to the longest and most fruitful love lives.

So what does this all mean? Well, it shows us how overwhelming and destructive stress can be. Do not think the job causes a man to have intimate problems. The cause is the way a particular job is performed. For example, being overly ambitious, a necessity to succeed, in one's opinion, can in reality become an obstacle instead of a tool for achievement. Of course it depends on how we measure success.

An injury is not done to a person who consents to it. Allegedly.

CHAPTER 6

Oh, What a Massage – Fun for Women

Intimate massage, just like any other kind of massage, has its own rules. It requires thorough theoretical knowledge, as well as hands-on practice. This massage, as its name implies, focuses on the intimate body parts. However, it does not mean it is solely limited to them. For example, one can combine certain elements of a relaxing massage or an erotic massage with an intimate one. It is also possible to simultaneously perform an intimate massage with another kind of massage. This happens when, for example, a masseuse uses one hand to massage a man's penis while massaging his chest, abdomen, etc., with the other hand. Such a combination of massage techniques done at the same time can also be performed by two masseuses.

Before beginning an intimate massage, it is best to take some time to start with relaxing and erotic massages. By doing so, one is able to create the right atmosphere, which ensures the patient's physical and psychological comfort. Eliminating nervous tension makes therapy much easier, so the time spent on creating a comfortable atmosphere is not in vain. This is the reason therapeutic intimate massage is also preceded by relaxing and erotic massages.

Intimate massage is a kind of massage that focuses on the intimate body parts, which in men include the:

- penis
- testicles
- scrotum—when massaging the testicles, one is also massaging the scrotum, but when massaging the scrotum one is not always in contact with the testicles
- crotch
- male G-spot

An intimate massage can be performed by:

- one or two masseuses
- more than two masseuses (in which case it is an intimate massage combined with another kind of massage, so it is not just purely an intimate massage. For example, it can be an intimate massage combined with a Chakra massage.)

An intimate massage can be performed:

- without any lubrication
- with the use of lubricants
- with the use of a baby powder

An intimate massage can be done with the use of different body parts:

- a hand or both hands
- a finger or multiple fingers

- fingertips
- breasts
- lips and tongue
- combining the use of mentioned and other body parts

Different accessories can be used during an intimate massage:

- one or more vibrators
- one or more brushes
- delicate fabrics such as flannel, silk, or velvet
- a towel or bed sheet
- beads
- a peacock feather
- others—be creative; use your imagination

A massage performed with the use of vibrators can be done one of two ways:

- directly—with the vibrator(s) touching the patient's skin
- indirectly—with the vibrator(s) taped to the outside of a hand or hands. This way the massage is performed with the hands, which are slightly vibrating.

The whole experience can also be enhanced through the use of other things:

- a stream of water
- hair
- a tubful of water (for an underwater massage)

Before going on to specific, intimate massage techniques. one should make sure to correctly differentiate between:

- the front of the penis, also known as the outer side of it
- the back of the penis, also called its inner side

The front of the penis is the side that is visible as the man stands in front of and facing you and the member is flaccid. It is important that the man is in a standing position when you are learning to identify the front and the back of the penis, because when lying down, either side of it can be visible—depending on its placement. It is important to be able to correctly discriminate the outer side of the member from the inner side because I will be referring to them throughout the book. So to reiterate, the front of the penis is its outer side and the back of the member is its inner side. When a man is lying down on his back with an erection, and you are standing in front of him, the back of his penis is visible.

As I've mentioned before, an intimate massage mainly includes the massage of a penis.

One must be able to distinguish several different parts of the organ:

- the trunk of the penis
- the tip, also called glans penis
- the base
- the part located under the skin of the crotch—which constitutes 40 percent of the length of the penis

An intimate massage can be performed regardless of the state of the member:

- flaccid
- a partial erection
- a full erection

An intimate massage can be alternated with an erotic or relaxing massage. This method is usually used when a man is very aroused. When that happens it is best to continue the massage but in less sensitive areas.

An intimate massage can be done in many ways, depending on the man's liking, but it is most important for the massage to be effective. This is why knowing many different techniques and presenting them to the patient is necessary. A technique can work for one person, while someone else would be completely indifferent to it. Observing a man's reactions will reliably show the most effective method for him. This is why one should combine different methods with the imagination in order to invent one's own original techniques.

Intimate massage for men can be divided into massaging:

- the whole penis, from the base to the tip
- the trunk of the penis from the base to the corona. The massage can include the whole trunk or its parts: outer, inner, or the sides.
- the base of the penis
- the tip
    o   through the foreskin
    o   with the foreskin retracted and with lubrication
- the frenulum of the prepuce (which is the most sensitive part of the penis)
    o   through the foreskin
    o   with the foreskin retracted and with lubrication
- the crotch, including the part of the penis located under the surface of the skin
- the groin
- the scrotum and testicles

Women who perform intimate massages without proper training usually use only a few techniques. They do not realize how much they and their partners are missing out on because there is an excess of different methods to choose from. I want to go over some. Knowing more than just a few brings great results. Those techniques can be used during a relaxing intimate massage just as well as during a therapeutic intimate massage.

A massage of a penis can be done in many different ways:

1. with the whole hand:
   a. gently, without applying any pressure
   b. with gentle pressure
   c. applying stronger pressure
   d. in one spot without moving the hand
2. with the fingertips
3. with the nails going with and against the grain
4. with the side of a hand
5. applying pressure with a thumb
6. using the fingers to stretch the member
7. stretching the penis with the use of a whole hand
8. using both hands simultaneously or alternating them
9. with a palm, using circular movements
10. along the length of the member
11. across the penis
12. with the lips
13. using the tongue
14. using the breasts
15. with or without lubrication
16. combining different methods

There are many more ways to perform a massage of the penis. I listed only some in order to give a general idea of the various possibilities. Do not deny yourselves the pleasure of using your priceless imagination.

The position of both the man and the masseuse during the massage can vary depending on the liking and creativity of both people. I will describe a few positions for men, but remember that there are many more and one can invent their own too. If you choose to try a position of your creation, remember to take into consideration your partner's approval and the position's functionality. It may seem that lying down is the only correct position because it is the most relaxing, but keep in mind that the goal of therapeutic intimate massage is to maintain arousal for a certain amount of time. Therefore, using different positions during the massage has its purpose. It can help to avoid reaching a level of arousal that is too high. It can also help to avoid monotony, which can, in turn, affect the sensations experienced during the massage. The right position can also enable two masseuses to perform the procedure simultaneously.

Usually during a massage a man takes one of the following positions:

- lying on his back
- sitting on his heels
- sitting up or propping himself up on his elbows
- standing up

The masseuse can do the massage in various positions as well. It is best to try as many positions as you can and observe your partner's reactions, which will enable you to easier control your partner's level of arousal.

Different positions a masseuse can assume during a massage:

1. When a man is lying on his back, you can:
   - sit on your heels in front of him or between his thighs. You can also sit on his thighs or straddle him while supporting yourself with your knees (so you are partially kneeling).
   - sit on either side, facing him
   - sit on either side, facing away from him
   - sit at his left or right with your body positioned perpendicular to him
   - sit behind him with your legs spread apart so that his head rests between your knees or thighs
   - sit behind him on your heels with his head resting on your thighs
   - lie on your side next to him
   - lie on top of him (use your breasts to massage him)
   - lie on your abdomen between his legs
2. When a man is sitting on his heels, you can:
   - sit in front of him
   - sit next to him
   - sit behind him
   - lie on your belly in front of him, propped up on your elbows with your head above his thighs
3. When a man is sitting down with his legs spread apart (he can also lean back to a half-sitting position and prop himself up with his elbows), you can:
   - sit in front of him
   - sit perpendicular to him
   - lie on your abdomen, between his thighs, propped up on your elbows

The man's position is similar to the one from the previous point, but the massage possibilities, and especially its effects, are different.

4. When a man is standing up, you can:
   - stand in front of him
   - stand behind him
   - stand to his side with your body perpendicular to him
   - sit in front of him on a bed or chair
   - sit on a chair or bed with your body perpendicular to him (facing his side; this position enables you to massage the penis with one hand and the testicles with the other, from behind)
   - kneel in front of him

Other positions are also available, but they are rarely used, so I will not describe them here.

Massaging the front and back of the member

Remember which side is the front, and which is the back of the penis, and while holding it in your hand rub either side of it. During such a massage, when a man is on his back, different techniques can be applied depending on your position.

There are a few different ways of holding a penis during a massage. Of course there are so many different methods of performing such a procedure that I will not even try to list them all. Instead, I will just focus on the four classic ways of holding a penis during a massage. They can be applied to an erect penis as well as a flaccid one. They are crucial tools of the trade. So, one should get to know and use them, and it will not take long to see results.

1. To massage the back of a member, sit in front of the man, slightly to his right (and perform the massage with your right hand), holding the penis in a classic way, meaning with your thumb grabbing its upper part.

2. To massage the front of the penis, position yourself exactly the same way as described in the previous point. The only difference is the position of the thumb, which should now be located at the base of the member. I recommend this method to all women, not just during a massage but also for fun and when trying to spice up foreplay.

3. To massage the front of the penis, but this time with the thumb around the tip of the member, sit to the left of the man, next to him, but not facing him, and use your right hand. This way your thumb is on the tip and your hand rubs the outer side of the penis.

4. Position yourself exactly the same way as described in the point above, but this time massage the back of the penis with your thumb around its base.

These distinctions are not just theoretical, they work well in practice. Sometimes even the smallest change in intimate stimulation can bring surprising results.

CHAPTER 7

Massaging a Flaccid Member

In this chapter I want to go over a few different methods of massaging a penis that is flaccid or partially erect. One can begin such a massage with gentle brushing of the genitals with the fingertips, the outside of a hand, or even the fingernails. When it comes to therapeutic intimate massage, it is not customary to use the hair, feet, or the whole body as tools, unless the patient requests it. Otherwise those body parts are usually reserved for relaxing intimate massages.

Intimate massage, just like any other type of massage, can be given and received in different positions. It is important to know them because they will become very handy in practice.

The basic positions of a man during massage:

- standing
- sitting
- sitting on his heels
- lying supine
- lying in a reclining position (leaning on his hands or elbows)

The most common massage techniques used on a flaccid or half-erect penis:

1. Classic massage—variant A (see: point 1 on page 70).
2. Classic massage—variant B (see: point 3 on page 70).
3. Inverted classic massage—a type of variant A (see: point 2 on page 70).
4. Inverted classic massage—a type of variant B (see: point 4 on page 70).
5. Massage the tip through the foreskin.
6. Twist the foreskin.
7. Retract and pull the foreskin back over the tip.
8. Squeeze the penis with your hand, gently at first and slowly increasing the pressure.
9. Do the same thing as in point 8, but this time squeeze the penis in different spots along the shaft several times and then do the same thing, using the other hand.
10. Stretch the foreskin in such a way that it extends over the tip of the member and then move it in all directions.
11. Stretch the foreskin just like above, but this time instead of moving it around, massage it between your thumb and index finger.
12. Stretch the foreskin so that it extends over the tip and then let it go. When you see the tip, repeat the action.
13. Massage the back of the penis as it rests in your hand. To do so, move your hand along the length of the member (all the way, until your fingers get between it and the testicles). You can also use circular movements.
14. While holding the penis in your hand, apply some pressure and move it up and down, to the sides or around in either direction.
15. While holding the member, alternate stretching it vertically and horizontally.

16. Gently tug on the penis.
17. Alternate gentle and stronger tugs.
18. While using a gentle grip, stretch the penis until it slips out of your hand.
19. Alternate both hands to stretch the penis. First, stretch it with one hand and when you feel that it is about to slip out, grab it with the other.
20. Using all your fingers (including your thumb), squeeze the member at its base.
21. Using all your fingers, squeeze the penis right below its tip.
22. Squeeze the tip through the foreskin.
23. Massage the tip through the foreskin in all directions.
24. The "Propeller"—spin the penis around its axis (the name of this technique comes from starting a plane engine, which in the early models had to be done by turning the propeller by hand).
25. Push the penis into its base and make circular movements.
26. Push the penis into its base and release your thumb. When the penis returns to its natural position repeat this method.
27. Using your fingers of one or both hands apply pressure around the base of the member.
28. Do the same thing as in the previous point, but around the shaft, just below the tip.
29. Pull the foreskin back and forth over the tip while holding the penis in your hand.
30. Press one of your fingers into the skin at the base of the penis. While doing so, you can try to get the foreskin to retract. When you succeed you can pull the foreskin back over the tip or you can continue the massage with the foreskin pulled back.

31. You can also try the previous technique with the use of more fingers, depending on your and your partner's preferences and the effectiveness of this method.
32. Toss the member up in your open palm.
33. Shake the penis while holding it at its base.
34. Shake the penis while holding it by its tip or by the foreskin stretched and extending over the tip.
35. Toss the penis from one hand to the other.
36. Grab the member with your fingers at its base and move them up the shaft. Repeat this motion several times.
37. Pull the foreskin back and forth over the tip, using the fingers of one hand.
38. Now do the same thing as above, but this time use both hands.
39. Squeeze the penis at its base, and without releasing the pressure, move your hand up toward the tip and release your grip. Then grab at the base and repeat.
40. Squeeze the penis at its base, and without releasing the pressure, move your hand up toward the tip and then back down.
41. Hold the penis at its base with one hand while using the other to massage the rest of it.
42. Hold the penis by its tip with one hand while using the other to massage the shaft and the base.
43. Using the palm of your hand pet the member, alternating between its front and back.
44. Place the member on the testicles and massage the genitals, using circular movements.
45. The "Dough"—place the penis between your palms and roll it back and forth like a piece of dough.
46. Massage the penis across instead of along its length, in a rolling motion:

    a. Place the penis on the man's abdomen and, using your palm, roll it back and forth.

    b. Massage the member with one hand as it rests on top of the other hand.

    c. Place the penis between your palms and move them to massage it.

47. Place the penis on the man's abdomen and, using circular movements, massage the back of it.

48. As the man lies on his back, put his penis on your palm. Now massage it with the other hand. You can also massage the back of it—just like in the previous point, with one exception: namely, the penis rests on your hand instead of the man's belly. The placement is similar, but the results may vary. So it is worth checking out both methods.

49. Using your open hand, stroke either the back or the front of the member in one direction.

50. This time move the hand back and forth on either side of the penis.

51. Now, move your hand or a finger along the member on its front and back.

52. Use your fingers, fingertips, or nails to move along the surface of the whole member.

53. Raise the penis to an upright/vertical position and let it go until it returns to its previous position, and then repeat the action several times.

54. Massage the area where the member meets the testes.

    a. Squeeze it.

    b. Use circular movements.

    c. Use your fingertips and nails to massage back and forth against the hair.

55. Grab the base of the penis along with the testicles with one hand and use the other to massage the shaft and tip in a random technique.

56. The "Throttle"—grab the penis on the front side with the thumb by either end of it (the base or the tip. You can change the position of your thumb during the massage). Move your wrist back and forth, just like you would with a throttle on a motorcycle, to increase or decrease the RPMs.

57. "Milk" the penis with one hand—grab it at its base and gently jerk it down.

58. "Milk" the penis just like in point 50, but this time, alternate both hands.

59. The "Pendulum"—when a man is standing, raise the member to one side and let it go. Next, repeat the procedure, but this time pick it up to the opposite side.

Massaging the frenulum is described in Chapter 8, which concerns an erect penis. However, there are a couple methods of massaging the frenulum when the penis is flaccid or partially erect.

Methods of stimulating the frenulum on a soft member:

1. Rubbing it with your finger through the foreskin (this cannot be done during an erection as the foreskin is pulled back).

2. Do the same as in the previous point, but this time use your nails.

3. Grab the foreskin between your forefinger and thumb where the frenulum is located and gently rub it.

Any other methods can be used regardless of the level of arousal.

CHAPTER 8

Massaging an Erect Penis

The positions of a man during a massage of an erect penis are exactly the same as the positions of a man during a massage of a flaccid one:

- standing up
- sitting down
- sitting on his heels
- half lying down (sitting back, propped up on his hands or elbows)
- lying down

The different techniques and methods of massage described below can and should be used with different positions because different sensations can be achieved with the same technique—but in a different position. For example, stimulating an erect member while a man is standing has a different effect from stimulating one when a man is lying down. When a man is standing during a massage, the effect is much stronger, as is the ejaculation—because in this position, the masseuse can bend the penis (not too much of course) and cause a much stronger ejaculation. Doing the same thing in a horizontal position, the ejaculation is weaker. So it is a good idea to try different methods in different positions.

The methods of massaging a penis, whether erect or flaccid, are often the same, but a man's reactions can differ depending on his level of arousal. This is why it is worth trying out the same techniques of massage during different levels of arousal.

There are no differences in the positions of the masseuse between the massage of a hard penis and a soft one. One can and should assume different positions during the massage for comfort and to observe a partner's reactions. A woman's body and her position surely has an effect on a man.

The positions one can assume during a massage have been described in the previous chapter, and everyone should freely experiment with them.

One can assume that massaging an erect penis is no different than massaging a flaccid one. It may seem so; however, the devil is in the details, and that is why it is important to pay attention to the differences. They can decide the massage's success (meaning its effectiveness). After all, the goal of a therapeutic intimate massage is to get rid of all ailments through the use of a group of compounds, endorphins, which naturally occur in every human body. In order for the healing process to be effective, one condition has to be met. The endorphins have to be produced for an appropriate period of time. If the massage is not attractive enough, the receiver of the massage is at risk of becoming bored and discouraged. It means a lack of effectiveness. In order to avoid such situations, switching both partners' positions often throughout the massage is recommended. Also, do not forget to use many different methods of massage during each session.

A variety of massage techniques and positions will ensure that boredom is not going to become one of the problems during a massage. Some may doubt that a man can become bored with his woman's efforts, but I assure that it is not only possible, but also that it happens in marriages of many years.

This book is supposed to help people rediscover the joy of intimate contact with a partner, to bring them closer together, and to help both enjoy life to its fullest. The technical information contained here is supposed to serve a specific, crucial goal, which should not manifest itself as a sign of exploitation or treating the other person like a sex object. As a matter of fact, it is designed to do just the opposite.

The art of massaging an erect penis:

1. Classic massage—variant A (see point 1 on page 70).
2. Classic massage—variant B (see point 3 on page 70).
3. Inverted classic massage—a type of variant A (see point 2 on page 70).
4. Inverted classic massage—a type of variant B (see point 4 on page 70).
5. The "Spring"—a classical variation. While the man is lying down, raise his erect member to a vertical position and let it go.
6. The "Sideways Spring"—the difference between this method and the previous one is that you bend the penis to the left or right instead of bringing it up.
7. The "Downward Spring"—in this variation of the spring, bend the member gently(!) past the vertical point.
8. The "Lemon Squeezer"—while the man is sitting or standing, put your palm on his erect penis and move it left and right as if you were squeezing the juice out of a

lemon. The man can also assume a lying position and then you have two options:

   a. perform the massage without raising the member to an upright position

   b. raise the member to a vertical position and then do "the lemon squeezer"

9. The "Screwdriver"—hold the penis like you would hold a screwdriver and alternate, turning it to the left and right.

10. The "Corkscrew"—grab the penis the same way as described in the previous exercise, but this time move your hand down the shaft to the base of the penis as if you were twisting the corkscrew onto the bottle. Next, "pull the cork out"—that is, grab the member in a tighter grip and move your hand upward toward the tip. While doing that you can simultaneously twist your hand to the left and right.

11. The "Reverse Corkscrew"—move your fingers from the middle of the penis toward its tip.

12. The "Indian Burn"—using both hands, twist the penis in opposite directions (just not too hard!).

13. The "Throttle"—hold the member by its outer side (with your thumb at either end of it, you can also switch the position of your thumb during the massage). While holding the penis, move your wrist back and forth like you would do with a throttle on a motorcycle.

14. The "Rolling pin"—this massage is performed across instead of along the penis

   a. massage the member with your palm as it rests on the man's abdomen

   b. place the penis on one hand and massage it with the other

   c. place the penis between your hands and massage it

15. The "Propeller"—spin the penis around its own axis (just like the first pilots would do with their planes' propellers to start engines).
16. The "Dough"—place the penis between your hands and roll it like you would roll some dough.
17. "Squeezing through the tunnel"—lube up your hand generously and make a fist, leaving some space in the middle so that you can slide it onto the tip, and then all the way down to the base. Your grip should be tight while allowing the penis to slide through.
18. "Catching the penis"—as the man is lying down, use one hand to bring the penis to an upright position and then let it go and catch it with your other hand.
19. Retract the foreskin and massage the tip with your open, lubed palm.
20. Lube your fingers and retract the foreskin. Massage the tip, the frenulum, and the corona with your fingers.
21. Massage the frenulum through the foreskin.
22. Massage the penis with one hand in one direction, from the base to the tip.
23. Do the same thing as in the previous exercise, but this time use your other hand to hold the testicles. You can also grab a part of the base as well.
24. This time massage the member with one hand in one direction from the tip to the base. This exercise requires a lot of lube.
25. Lube up one of your hands and use it to massage the penis back and forth while using your other hand to keep the foreskin pulled back by holding the scrotum.
26. Do the same thing as in the point above, but this time, do not hold the scrotum.

27. Lube up your hand and massage the penis in one direction from the tip to the base. You can also include the testes in the massage.
28. Stretch the penis in one direction from the base to the tip. This exercise can be performed:
    a. without lube
    b. with lube
29. You can hold the penis one of two ways during a massage:
    a. with the under grip
    b. with the over grip
30. Using the fingers of both hands, simultaneously massage both sides of the penis or its front and back. To do so you can use:
    a. a plane motion
    b. circular movements
31. This method requires you to combine two types of movements at the same time. As you move your hand along the length of the member, try to also employ a rolling or circular movement across it.
32. Alternate both hands to massage the penis from its tip to the base. This creates a strong sensation, which can lead to an ejaculation. When using this technique always remember to lube up the member, especially at the tip. To make this exercise more interesting, instead of ending the downward motion of your hand at the base of the member you can extend it to the testicles.
33. Use both hands alternately to massage the penis from the base up, gently stretching it, while gradually increasing the strength of the pull. Your partner may experience different sensations depending on the direction of the massage and whether it is done horizontally or vertically.
34. Use the edge of your hand to massage the area where the base of the penis meets the abdomen.

35. Massage the part of the penis which is hidden from view, just underneath the skin of the crotch.
36. Squeeze the member with your hand:
    a. in one place
    b. along its length
37. Alternate both hands to massage the penis from the base up, then switch directions from top to bottom. After a series of movements of one kind switch back to the other.
38. Stretching through the hoops:
    a. start with both hands holding the penis; one in the area where the balls meet the shaft and the other right above the base. Then, slowly move the hand above the base towards the tip, while stretching the member, at the same time
    b. grab the penis with both hands, so that they meet around its middle, and pull them away from each other
39. Use one hand to hold the tip of the penis while massaging it with the other, from its middle down.
40. Using your finger or fingers, apply pressure to the base of the penis. While doing so, you can cause the foreskin to:
    a. stay covered over the tip
    b. get pulled back from the tip
41. Stretch the penis while simultaneously bending it in different directions.
42. Gently move your fingers along the length of the penis, starting with the testes:
    a. working your way up and then repeating the motion
    b. to the tip and then back down
43. Using your fingers, apply pressure to the area where the penis meets the testicles.

44. As the man is lying on his back, start the massage along the abdomen towards the member, and then move on the shaft until it reaches a vertical position. Then, allow the penis to return to its original position and slide your hand down the other side including the testicles. Keep repeating the process over again.

Massaging the frenulum

The frenulum is the most sensitive body part of a man. It takes up a very small surface area, but it plays an exceptional role in the stimulation process. It is located on the back of the penis, about an inch below the tip.

Massaging the frenulum can be done:

- with your fingertip or nail (through the foreskin)
- with your tongue
- with your lips
- with a nipple
- with different accessories, such as:
  o a vibrator
  o a brush
  o whatever your imagination can come up with

How to massage the frenulum:

1. A "punctual massage" is based on repeating multiple, short-lived impulses. It can be performed with your finger, tongue, vibrator, etc.
2. Circular movements are often used during oral massages. This type of stimulation is performed with your tongue, both when the penis is in your mouth and when it is

not. However, these movements do not always have to be circular, they can also be done along and across the frenulum. The sensations created by this type of stimulation are highly recommended.

3. Tapping it with the fingers is a very interesting method.
4. Massaging "against the grain"—done with the smooth part of your nail.
5. "Sucking it in" with your lips.

The frenulum can be touched:

- indirectly through the foreskin (most often)
- directly (usually requires a lot of lubrication)

Coming in contact with the frenulum can be done:

- without lubrication
- with lubrication

CHAPTER 9

Testicle Massage

The positions assumed by a man during a testicle massage are very similar to those applied during a massage of a penis, but they are not exactly the same. They are as follows:

- lying down
- sitting on the heels
- half sitting up (propped up on his elbows or hands)
- standing up

As far as the masseuse goes, she can use the same positions that one would use during a massage of the penis, described in Chapter 6.

Testicle massage and scrotum massage are terms that are oftentimes used interchangeably. The difference between the two is that sometimes—actually, very seldom—the scrotum gets massaged, without the testicles being touched at all. Only when the scrotum gets stretched, so that the testicles move up or down, a scrotum massage is possible, whereas, a testicle massage is always performed through the scrotum, because there is no other possibility.

The art of testicle massage

1. Use circular movements to massage the whole surface of the testicles.
2. Alternate both hands to massage them from the bottom up.
3. Do the same as above but in the opposite direction.
4. Do the same as above but starting from the groin.
5. Stroke testicles only in one direction using one hand.
6. Hold the penis in one hand and move the fingers of your other hand along the testicles, starting from the penis down. Repeat this movement many times, changing the position of your fingers, so the massage includes the whole surface of the scrotum.
7. Do the same thing as described in the previous point, but this time, change the direction of the massage (from the crotch up).
8. Do the same thing as above, but this time alternate the direction of the massage with each stroke.
9. Pull the scrotum.
10. Stretch the scrotum down by one hand.
11. Alternate both hands in stretching the scrotum in different directions.
12. Pull the scrotum to the sides.
13. Twist the scrotum.
14. Gently tug at the testicles.
15. "Toss" the testicles from hand to hand.
16. Stretch the penis and the testicles in the same direction.
17. Simultaneously stretch the penis upwards and the testicles in the opposite direction
18. Using one hand, massage the member and the testicles, alternating the direction of the massage.

19. Using your fingertips, gently massage around the testicles.
20. Gently squeeze the testes with your whole hand.
21. Raise the testicles with your hand and then let them drop to their original position.
22. Put the testes in your hand and move them in every direction: raise them, pull them down, pull them horizontally and to the sides, spin the scrotum to the left and to the right.
23. Hold the testicles in your hand and pull them to make the member raise up.
24. Make circular movements with your palm all over the testes.
25. Use a plane motion to massage across the testicles with your palm.
26. Massage the bottom of the testicles as you raise them, after you let them drop massage the front of them, applying gentle pressure.
27. Using your fingertips, massage the bottom of the scrotum.
28. Do the same thing as above, but use your fingers to tap the scrotum this time.
29. Tap the outer side of the scrotum with your fingers while moving them either up or down its surface.
30. Move your fingertips down the testicles and when you get to the bottom switch directions and move back up, using your nails instead of your fingertips.
31. Using the fingers of both your hands, massage the sides of the scrotum while gently pulling on them.
32. Massage the front side of the scrotum in a downward motion, while holding the member with your other hand or with your lips.
33. Grab the scrotum between the testicles and stretch it.

34. Use the fingers of both your hands to gently pull both of the testicles.

35. When the man has an erection and is in a lying position, pull the scrotum quickly and rhythmically but gently, causing the penis to come up to a vertical position and drop back down.

36. Sit behind your partner and alternate both hands to massage the testes from the crotch up.

37. This time, sit down facing your man and alternate using both your hands to massage the testicles from the penis down to the crotch.

38. Lie down next to your partner and raise the testicles and let them go. Next, stretch them in opposite direction.

39. Assume the same position as in the previous point, but this time place your fingertips where the penis meets the scrotum. Move the testicles (without touching them) by bending and straightening your fingers.

40. Once again use the same position as in the previous two points, but place your hand a bit lower this time, so that you can stimulate the crotch and the bottom of the scrotum. When you bend your fingers, use your fingernails to massage those areas and when you straighten them, use your fingertips.

Massaging the crotch and the groin

This is a very important erogenous zone that is often neglected in foreplay but absolutely cannot be treated this way during an intimate massage. Sometimes this area is stimulated by fingers during an oral massage of the penis. There are not many techniques to choose from, but they definitely bring about unforgettable experiences.

How to massage the crotch and groin

1. Place your hand on your man's thigh and move your fingertips up along one side of the groin. After repeating that motion back and forth a few times, move to the other side of the groin through the crotch.
2. Place your hand on the testicles and use your fingertips to stimulate the groin. This method allows you to simultaneously stimulate two erogenous zones (even three if you are using oral massage).
3. Place your hand under the testicles in such a way that you touch both sides of the groin simultaneously, one with your thumb, and the other with your index and middle fingers, with the rest of the fingers touching the crotch. Additionally, when stimulating the groin, use the side of your hand to rub the bottom of the testicles.
4. Place your hand on the testicles in a way that your thumb and other fingers touch both sides of the groin at the same time. Then, massage along the groin.
5. Using your fingertips, stimulate the surface of the crotch with:
   a. circular movements
   b. movements across the crotch
   c. movements along the crotch
6. Spread your fingers and place them on the outer edges of the crotch, and then move them in until they meet and then back out. Repeat this motion many times.
7. Place your hand on the testicles in a way that will allow you to massage the crotch with your fingers. For this exercise you can use circular or plane movements. Remember that you can also use your fingernails. If you do it skillfully, it can lead to greater amounts of pleasure.

CHAPTER 10

As Hard as a Rock . . . and Other Exercises

I assume that at this point in the book you have already mastered the basic massage techniques and are ready to move on to more advanced exercises, which will allow you to enjoy intimate moments for longer period of time and in more ways.

Exercise: the plateau phase

The plateau phase on the "sexual bliss scale" is characterized by a high level of excitement. This is when the erection gets very hard and the penis gets darker in color. At this time the penis may also excrete pre-ejaculation fluid. The plateau phase is followed by an orgasm. It is up to the individual, for the most part, how long one can enjoy the strong arousal of the plateau phase. When doing the exercises described below, do not just focus on your own pleasure but remember your partner. Do not try to use all of the methods at once; instead, spread them out over a few days.

1. This exercise is supposed to allow one to experience the plateau on a few different levels of arousal, just by changing the rhythm of breathing, which will enable to stay on each level three to five minutes. Have your woman caress the front of your body until you feel relaxed, after which she can proceed to stimulate your genitals. Focus on the sensations and your breathing. When you feel your arousal reaching a higher level, slow down your breathing and try to remain at that level. When you feel your excitement dropping, quicken your breath again.

2. This exercise is based on hip movements. Use them in a way similar to the breathing technique from the previous exercise. It is also designed to help you stay at a specific level of arousal. Move your hips in circular and thrusting movements to raise your level of excitement. Start the sensual movements when you feel your arousal decreasing and then add some verve to climb to the subsequent levels. Another variation of this exercise is to combine those hip movements with Kegel muscle exercises. This way you can lower your level of arousal with the Kegel muscles and raise it with your hip muscles.

3. This is one of those exercises where the lack of concentration is actually a good thing. Sounds mysterious? Here is how it works. Have your partner stimulate your genitals with her hand or mouth. When you feel the climax approaching, turn your attention away from the stimulated area and toward something else. Your level of arousal should slightly decrease. To increase your arousal, focus on the stimulated area once again.

This exercise will allow you to last in a blissful state—on the border of an orgasm—even for a few minutes.

As hard as a rock

The plan described below is supposed to help you reach really satisfying erections. The stages of that plan are as follows:

- the initiation—happens in your head when you feel aroused
- the filling out—the penis becomes thicker and longer because of increased blood flow
- the stiffening—the member becomes hard caused by the closing of the valves, which block off the flow of blood
- maintaining the erection—the ability to keep up the erection for a specific amount of time

Exercise: how to attain a quicker erection

If you are worried that achieving an erection takes too long, this is a perfect exercise to start with. Its purpose is to cause an erection through a large amount of blood flowing to the penis. After a suitable amount of time (about two months), you will notice that your erection is fuller and that you are attaining it quicker than before. You can train alone or with your partner.

All you need for this exercise is about five minutes. Have your partner lube up her hand and slowly caress the base of your penis, occasionally squeezing the shaft harder. Since this is not masturbation it is important for the movements to be calm and balanced.

Exercise: relaxing the Kegel muscle

Men often make the mistake of thinking that squeezing the Kegel muscle allows them to increase their erection. Unfortunately, if you repeat this procedure often, you will see that reaching an erection will take longer than usual.

If you have developed the bad habit of contracting the Kegel muscle at the wrong time, this exercise will help you get rid of it. Start with orally massaging your woman and then rest for a while. Next, lie on your back and let your partner stimulate you orally and with her hand. When she feels that you are squeezing your Kegel, she should stop and let you know about it. Let her resume the massage when you feel relaxed again. As she lets you know about each unwanted contraction, your self-control instinct should allow you to get rid of the habit.

Exercise: when your arousal and erection do not go hand-in-hand

Surely it seems logical that an erection grows proportionally to the increase of arousal, which means that the member should reach its hardest point right before an orgasm. However, that is not always the case, and you may feel disappointed that your penis is not keeping up. So how can you make your erection grow with your arousal?

You may not be able to get your penis to catch up to your level of arousal, but you can learn to control your arousal until it levels off with your erection. Take into consideration that arousal decreases faster than an erection. So, next time you climax, pay attention to how fast your erection decreases in relation to the fall of your level of arousal.

Start out with your partner stimulating you orally. When you feel your arousal increasing but your erection is not keeping up with it, ask your woman to slow down until both the arousal and the erection level off. Resume the exercise and be in control of the situation the whole time. Do not get discouraged if you are not able to synchronize your erection with your arousal on the higher levels at first. Instead, repeat the exercise until you learn how to gain control over the situation.

There is another variation of this exercise that makes you the active party, enabling you to control what happens to you, because you know what excites you. Rub your member against your woman's genitalia, move in a way that excites you, and when you feel that your arousal is getting ahead of your erection, stop the activity.

Exercise: In search of the lost erection

Some men harm themselves with false beliefs. For example, they think that when being one on one with a woman their erection should be constantly full and hard. However, it is normal for the erection to fluctuate throughout the sexual encounter. If you feel your member getting soft, the worst thing you can do is to squeeze its muscles. If you do that, you can be sure that it will get even softer, so relax and focus on the pleasant sensations.

For this exercise you need twenty minutes and an understanding partner. To make her even more understanding, give her some pleasure, caress her body, stimulate her orally, etc., before you start the exercise. Then, lie on your back and let her take care of you. Give yourself fully to her; let her play with your penis and testicles as she wants before she begins oral stimulation. When your penis grows visibly, stop the stimulation, even if you want to go on, until you reach the lowest level of erection and then resume the exercise again. The idea here is to reach a higher level of erection than previously. In the twenty minutes allotted for this exercise you can attain and lose the erection (only to regain it, and perhaps reach a higher level) several times.

After performing this exercise you will see that you can gain an erection even if your partner is not stimulating you, but if that does not happen right away, do not stress out. It is just a sign that you are too tense. Perhaps another session the next day will allow you to relax to the point where attaining an erection will not be a problem.

Exercise: another way to perform an oral massage

If you have a problem with keeping up an erection, this exercise will provide the proper stimulation, especially at the higher levels of arousal.

Your partner should perform the massage in a way that is exceptionally exciting to you and will bring you to a high level of arousal. Up to this point you are the passive side, but once you reach a high level of arousal, switch positions with your woman so that she is lying down, with you kneeling over her. You should position yourself in a way that will let you have easy access to her mouth while being comfortable at the same time, since you will be in this position from a few to a dozen or so minutes. When you kneel in a position that meets these criteria, hold your penis in your hand, caress your partner's lips with it, and slide it into her mouth from time to time. Occasionally your woman can take control and lick and suck your member for some time and then become the passive side again.

A satisfying orgasm and ejaculation

Adult males often face the problem of decreased sensitivity to sexual stimuli, meaning they need to be strongly aroused to feel satisfied with sex. What causes such a problem? It can stem from a routine, monotony in the bedroom, or even bad habits during masturbation, which can cause the member to become less sensitive. If someone has not had sexual relations with a woman for a long time, perhaps he got used to strong or even brutal stimulation. Then, when that person gets together with a woman, he may feel that the sensations created by her touch or by penetrating her body are too subtle and inadequate to reach an orgasm.

Another reason that can be attributed to decreased sensitivity of the penis is too much time spent on masturbation. There is no norm that would regulate the appropriate amount of time one should spend on masturbating. Some people need only a few minutes while others require more time. However, if you spend a half an hour or more on this activity, start shortening that amount. At first make it shorter by five minutes, and then the following week take off another five and so on, until you can be satisfied with ten to fifteen minutes of touching yourself. Yet another reason for a lack of or diminished satisfaction with the sexual relations with your partner may be too frequent masturbation. It does not mean you should feel remorse or that you are doing something wrong. It only means you have to learn to increase your sensitivity to stimuli.

Exercise: sensitive to new sensations

Your mission during this exercise is to learn to masturbate in a more gentle manner. "More gentle" means slower and with less force, but without compromising the strength of the orgasm.

You will need fifteen to twenty minutes for this exercise. Start masturbating in a way that you normally do. After a while slow down your movements a bit, and then do so after a minute or even more, and so on. You should realize that what you are doing is more like gentle caressing, which would take place between you and your partner, rather than intensive masturbation like you got used to without one. If at first you notice having problems with maintaining your arousal, alternate the intense moves with more subtle ones, and with each session add more and more gentle moves and caressing until you realize that you practically do not need strong stimulation.

CHAPTER 11

Tradition of Oral Massage

This subject is often controversial and is met with resistance from many people. However, the contact of one's lips with a partner's intimate areas is really quite natural. Perhaps it takes getting used, but it is definitely worth the effort. This experience is surely one of the most erotic. Of course such massage only makes sense when both sides want it, but it is really worth a try in order not to hastily deprive oneself of one of the biggest intimate pleasures.

The oral massage of a man

I will start with a quick lesson on penile anatomy. Many women probably don't even think about it, but this knowledge can be helpful. Consequently, it can intensify the healing impact. The first thing that is noticeable about a penis is the foreskin (or lack thereof). Circumcision has its pros and cons but this is not the time or place to discuss the matter. For now, let's take a look at the stem* of the penis. At its top there is an oval ending, which is a bit bigger in diameter than the stem, informally known as the head and also known as the tip, which is connected to the rest of the penis by the corona.* The small fold of skin connecting the foreskin with the tip is called the frenulum. It is located on the back side of the penis and is very sensitive to touch. The frenulum, when stimulated with the tongue, is sure to bring a man to ecstasy. Unfortunately, this part of the male anatomy is usually removed during circumcision. Below the tip is the stem of the member, which does not have a lot of nerve endings, meaning that if one focuses all the caressing on this area, miracles should not be expected. Located below the stem is the scrotum, which looks like a sack, and it contains testicles, where the sperm is produced. Skillful stimulation of this area can bring a lot of pleasure, or at least intensify the sensations created by caressing the penis. There is one more important spot on the map of male erogenous zones: the "little lips" on the top of the head of the member called the urethra, where the sperm is ejaculated from. This is not a medical textbook so I am not going to go into more details. Now that the theory has been presented, it is time for some hands on.

Lesson #1

Start with a full body relaxing massage, and then proceed to caressing the genitals. Keep at it for as long as you need until both of you are completely relaxed. Next, begin moving your lips and tongue slowly along your partner's thighs, testicles, and penis. You can try touching the bottom of his testes with your lips and then slide your tongue between his thighs and sack. Explore different areas of his body with your lips and tongue and watch his reaction to your movements. Put his penis in your mouth and then slowly slide it out. Remember that neither of you should feel forced to do anything, and you should primarily listen to your instincts. The goal here is not to cause an orgasm but to learn to enjoy the intimate oral contact with your loved one's genitals. Use only your lips and tongue and remember to relax your tongue. If you feel your tongue stiffening, switch positions.

Under no circumstances should you let this exercise be dictated by ambition. If you notice you are starting to worry if your caressing is satisfying your partner, take a break and return to massaging other parts of his body.

Remember that this is supposed to be an oral massage, so try not to use your hands. Focus only on the sensations created with your tongue and lips. One more important thing: no biting is allowed at this time. This area of the body is so sensitive that even a gentle bite can cause pain and then all the effort goes to waste.

Side note

Since oral stimulation is one of the most satisfying sexual experiences for men, it is possible—even very probable—that stimulating his penis with your lips will cause an orgasm. This is where a problem arises for many women because some get repulsed even at the thought of an ejaculation in their mouth. In such a situation you can finish the massage "outside." If you do not have such reservations but don't want to swallow the semen, you can discretely spit it out. The best scenario in a man's eyes is for a woman to swallow, but don't do anything against your will. However, it is worth to take a minute to think about why you have such a reservation. Conceivably at some point you may decide that you want to overcome it and maybe you will be able to do so without much trouble. Not every woman will consider the taste of sperm to be great or even neutral for that matter, but trying it in small amounts at first and then "upping the dose" will help you get used to this kind of experience and perhaps even like it.

If you want to begin with small amounts of semen, start with oral sex soon after your man has ejaculated. You can also try to place your tongue on top of the penis right before the ejaculation. If you can do it in time, the seed will just run down the bottom of your tongue. Another method is to rub the member on the inside of your cheek, in the very last stage of the oral massage so that the sperm lands there and not down your throat. In reality there is a small possibility of that happening if you do not put the member deep into your mouth. Probably it will not happen if you are just starting to experiment with this massage technique.

Lesson #2

If you think you have successfully completed the first lesson and can now touch your partner's genitals with your mouth without any reservations, and perhaps with pleasure, it is time to move on. Fellatio can be a really beneficial influence on your lover. If his erection problems are caused by stress related to a necessity of proving himself as a perfect lover, this form of intimacy will allow him to relax and fully surrender himself to you (and your lips . . .). Fellatio is a Latin term meaning "oral sex," during which the man is the passive and the woman the active party. During fellatio a penis is kissed, licked, and sucked, and here is how to do it:

1. With one hand, hold the stem of the penis and bend it in different directions to gain access to all its different parts, especially the tip. Make circular movements with your tongue, gently stimulating the corona.
2. Move the tip of your tongue along the seam of the member toward the frenulum. Pull the foreskin back over the tip with your tongue and then stimulate it with gentle vibrating moves.
3. Open your mouth and grab the tip of the penis with your lips (be careful not to use your teeth!).

4. Move your lips up and down the shaft, gently at first, and then gradually increase the pressure of your lips on the penis. Slide the member as far into your mouth as is comfortable for you. Your partner can grab your head and steer your movements, but both of you should be careful to not insert the penis too deep and choke you.

The technique of "deep-throating" is for the more experienced. It is best to avoid unwanted complications. In case of uncircumcised men, one should be careful when retracting the foreskin without any lubrication as it can be painful (although it usually shouldn't prove to be). It is good for the penis to be moist either from saliva or pre-cum. A few moves back and forth with your mouth over the tip should do the trick.

It is, of course, just a general outline of a scenario that should be diversified by both partners and developed to each other's liking. For example, caressing of the testicles is very much underappreciated. When performing this activity, one should suck and lick with special care and intuition since this area is prone to pain. Some men also enjoy the stimulation of the perineum—a small area between the testes and the anus.

When choosing a position, a big factor is the imagination. It is important for both partners to feel comfortable. However, if a woman wants to make her man feel really special, she should kneel in front of him when he is standing and grab his hips. This way she is treating him to a real visual feast, and even though he may think that he is the master of the situation, all the control lies upon her.

If that position seems uncomfortable, there are other options, such as kneeling between the partner's legs as he is lying down, or perhaps lying across his body. The woman can, if she prefers a more passive position, lie on her back and have her partner kneel over her chest.

These are just some of the basic positions, but some things should always be considered no matter what the arrangement of the bodies is. First, all positions can be freely modified with the use of the imagination; and secondly, one must always remember that the purpose here is an oral massage that is as positively influencing as it is satisfying, not some acrobatics.

Side note

There are many different ways to make an oral massage better with certain accessories. For instance, placing an ice cube in the mouth and kissing the penis works well. A refreshing experience is also guaranteed by placing a piece of gum in the mouth or taking a sip of cold champagne right before the start of the massage. If there are no useful accessories nearby, one can rinse her mouth, according to his liking, with really cold or warm water to diversify the experience.

Even though fellatio is colloquially referred to as "sucking a penis," in reality it has nearly nothing to do with that activity. Sucking arouses a man greatly, but in some cases it can cause pain. Although a penis can be actually sucked, for a short time and really gently, a woman should focus on putting the tip of the penis in and out of her mouth, on caressing it with her lips and moving her tongue all over it, including the corona and the frenulum.

The penis is the most sensitive erogenous zone. Teasing the foreskin with the tip of the tongue causes outstanding arousal in a man. In general, oral stimulation for most men is a really delightful experience. The glans penis, located at the end of the member is unusually sensitive and therefore susceptible to pleasure from such caressing. Massaging the tip requires certain caution as to not cause any pain.

Many men like when a woman rapidly moves her tongue across the penis. After gaining some experience, this can be achieved even without placing the glans penis in the mouth. It is such a strong sensation that a man can lose his orientation. A woman can also suck and lick the testicles. When doing so one must be very careful, since the testes are unusually sensitive, and even though a man can experience much pleasure when the sack seems to be separating from the crotch, it can also cause pain. It is not recommended to place both testicles in the mouth because one can unintentionally cause pain due to a sudden spike in arousal or loss of control. One can also try licking and gently biting the small area between the testicles and the anus, called the perineum. It is in this region that the male G-spot is located.

Lesson #3

A known Hindu text, probably created in the first century BC, known as the *Kama Sutra*, offers some advice on oral sex. It is worth learning, testing, and applying the knowledge of the ancient people in this matter. Learning sexual tricks of antiquity can stimulate one's imagination to create new ones for the needs of today's lovers. The importance of those new ideas is that they are one's own.

Here is what the early civilized people recommend when it came to oral stimulation of a penis:

1. This method (can be classified as the classic technique) is performed by holding the penis in one hand while

squeezing with the lips as they move up and down the shaft.

2. Biting—should be done by grabbing the tip of the penis with all the fingers and squeezing the sides with the lips or even teeth (very carefully!).

3. Stretching—is accomplished by placing the tip of the member in one's mouth and having her squeeze her lips around it and pull her head back until it slips out. Then the process should be repeated.

4. Squeezing—the lips squeeze around the member as it is inserted into her mouth. Next, the penis is taken out and reinserted in the same manner as before.

5. Sucking in—the penis is placed between her lips, which grab it, and then she sucks it inside.

6. Licking—skimming the penis with the tongue, from the base to the tip.

7. Sucking—about half the penis is placed inside her mouth so she can suck it passionately. It is done correctly if she feels her cheeks getting sucked in during this activity.

8. Swallowing—it is done by inserting the entire penis into her mouth and squeezing it with the throat, as if intending on swallowing it.

The aforementioned oral stimulation techniques are for committed couples and are not necessarily an element of therapeutic intimate massage. This book is designated not only for people with experience in this domain but also for those who wish to gain such experience. There are many women who would like to take care of their men in this way, but their problem is that they lack practice. They are afraid of being awkward and give up. In reality, the women only need to know how to start, and their partners will not even suspect they do not have much skill. Just the fact that a woman accepts this form of stimulation and her willingness to perform it should delight her partner. With time, these bedroom antics can transform into a form of oral massage used for therapeutic or preventive measures.

<u>Lesson #4</u>

Here are a few suggestions, especially for beginners. It is worth trying them out, while remembering that the imagination and its ingenuity take priority:

1. The man is positioned on his back with the woman bent over his penis or with her head on his abdomen. At first she kisses the penis and touches it with her tongue without taking it into her mouth. When accustomed to this experience she slowly engulfs it in her lips. This should be done while holding the member in her hand as to have control of its reactions. These reactions are slight movements that may occur when a penis is erect, and they include trembling and rising of the penis. This often happens when one's partner provides him with especially great stimulation, such as licking his frenulum. At first the contact between the lips and the penis can be seemingly insignificant. It is better to focus more on stimulating the glans penis as well as the shaft, especially its inner side, with the tongue.

   The positions of the bodies should be determined by women because oftentimes they do not wish their partners to see what they are doing. This happens when a woman is uncertain about her skills.

2. Once again the man lies supine as the woman moves her hand along the inner side of his penis, from the base up to the tip, watching it "jerk up" as she nears the

frenulum. Then she substitutes the hand for her tongue as she continues observing the member's reactions.

3. After the first experiences with the *French love*, it is time to take some bolder steps, meaning inserting the whole glans penis into the mouth. Next, the penis should be placed even farther into her mouth, but without forcing anything. It should be done with ease, almost effortlessly. To achieve that, one can and should try the techniques described here.

4. It is a good idea for beginners who do not want their partners to see what they are doing to assume the "69 position".* It allows both to concentrate on what they are doing instead of on each other and leaves much room for experimentation and fun.

5. This exercise is very simple: the woman places the penis in her mouth and holds it there while massaging the penis and testicles with her hand.

6. This time, while holding the member in her mouth, the woman bends it in different directions. When doing that, one should remember to move the member with her mouth and not to massage it with her lips.

7. Inserting and taking the penis out of her mouth, waiting a few seconds and reinserting can be exciting for both.

8. At this stage it is time to learn how to suck. The first step is to draw and relax the cheeks. After repeating that a few times one adds a finger to the equation. When practicing on her finger, she can imagine that it is a penis and therefore gain some practice and confidence. Then, when it is time to do it to her partner, he will surely express admiration and delight.

9. This exercise is very similar to the previous one with one important modification. Instead of putting a finger in

her mouth, she places the tip between her lips and sucks until it slips in.

10. At this point no one should feel awkward when performing an oral massage and it should be fine to have her partner watch. In this exercise the woman positions herself on her back, with her partner kneeling over her. In this position she stimulates her partner's glans penis. If the member is flaccid she sucks it in, but when it is erect she puts her lips around it and uses her tongue to lick the:
    a. area around the glans penis
    b. frenulum
    c. tip of the penis

11. The man stands as the woman kneeling in front of him places his member in her mouth and then bends it to a horizontal position. After stimulating it for some time she bends the penis even farther down, using her hand for help if necessary. It is extremely crucial to remember to do it slowly for the first time and to discuss with one's partner how far down his penis can be bent without hurting him. Every man is different and so is his sensitivity and range of motion.

12. This time the man sits on a bed while the woman kneels in front of him on the floor. She takes his flaccid penis into her mouth and squeezes with her lips right below the glans penis. Then she pulls the member by tilting her head back as far as she can.

13. The combination of oral massage and the so-called "fingering" brings men incredible sensations. The woman sucks the penis while moving her thumb and index finger along the blood vessels that run along its inner side. Next, she moves the same fingers below the scrotum, and using the same motion rubs that area while simultaneously moving the rest of the finger up and down his testicles.

These moves are somewhat similar to milking a cow and cause an intense orgasm.

14. In this exercise the woman rests on her back with her head on a pillow. The man kneels above her at such an angle that she can easily grab his penis with her lips without using her hands. The movements are done by the man, who must control his thrust in order not to go any deeper than his partner deems acceptable.

Oral massage has significant meaning to many people, both men and women. It creates much excitement, but that is not all. Skillfully dosed, it can be used as an element of the love game, and also applied to therapeutic intimate massage. It is obvious that it is important to the cohesion of a relationship (a relationship in where partners like these types of activities). Oral massage also plays a lead role in the relaxing intimate massage, so it is worth systematizing the knowledge on this subject. Later it will be easier to take advantage of it during mutual exercises and it sure will be more fun.

Oral massage is performed with the help of:

- lips
- tongue
- lips and tongue in simultaneous stimulation
- inner cheeks
- teeth (very rarely and with much caution)

It can be done:

- through the foreskin
- with the foreskin retracted, so there is direct contact between the glans penis and the mouth

- along the whole area of the member from its base all the way to its tip

Types of movements

1. Lips:
   a. massaging the glans penis with the lips
   b. sucking (the tip of the penis while squeezing it with the lips right below the corona)
   c. rolling the foreskin back (and pulling it back over the tip with the use of the lips or fingers)
   d. sucking the penis into the mouth
   e. rhythmically squeezing the glans penis or shaft with the lips
   f. rhythmically squeezing the penis with the lips while moving along its length between the tip and the base.
   g. squeezing the glans penis with the lips through the foreskin
2. Tongue:
   a. stimulation of the area where the foreskin meets the glans penis
   b. stimulation of the tip with the foreskin pulled back
   c. stimulation of the frenulum:
      - with circular movements
      - along its length (back and forth or just in one direction)
      - across it
      - punctual massage
3. Inner cheeks.
4. Teeth (only through the foreskin)

The man's positions when receiving an oral massage:

a. standing
b. lying
c. sitting
d. sitting on one's heels

The woman's positions while giving an oral massage:

- sitting or kneeling
- lying supine
- lying on her abdomen, next to her partner, or between his legs
- lying on her side
- "on all fours" in front of her partner
- "on all fours" behind her partner (to be more precise, partially behind him and partially over him)

All this seems obvious, but in practice a woman who does not have any professional training uses one, maybe two types of oral stimulation. How is she to help her partner who has, for example, erectile dysfunction, with such limited skills?

The art of giving oral massage to men

1. One takes the penis into her mouth and massages it back and forth without removing it.
2. The woman places the member in her mouth and massages it to let it slip out after a while. Then she reinserts and continues.
3. She retracts the foreskin with her lips and then tries to pull it back over the tip, also in the same manner.
4. The woman rolls the foreskin back with the use of her lips and then, with her fingers, returns it to its original state. Then she repeats the massage.

5. As the woman keeps the penis in her mouth, the partner moves it around.

6. She lies on her abdomen in front of her partner and in that position stimulates him using the methods described in points 7-15. Of course these techniques can also be applied to different positions of both partners, but it is highly recommended to try them, especially when using this one.

7. The woman slides her mouth on to the penis using three different speeds, each time placing the member deeper into her mouth. There are two variations:
   a. the woman returns to the starting point each time
   b. she continues without returning to the beginning

8. One uses her lips to make circular movements all over the penis.

9. With the member in her mouth the woman moves her head to the left and right, slightly at first and then increases the angle of the bending.

10. The woman places the penis in her mouth and (slowly!) pulls it down as far as it will go.

11. After placing the member between her lips, she massages the frenulum and the glans penis with her tongue.

12. She does the same thing here without putting the penis in her mouth.

13. This time she picks a random oral massage while simultaneously touching the testes with her hand(s).

14. One places the member in her mouth but does not put her lips around it. She moves her head sideways, back and forth and around. She uses the inside of her cheeks for stimulation. It is a specific kind of touch and is worth experiencing, especially when the penis is erect.

15. She can also try performing the same actions as in the previous exercise but on a flaccid member.

16. The woman can use her lips to squeeze the penis.
17. One can rinse her mouth with cold water prior to starting the massage.
18. Warm water can also be used.
19. The woman places as much of the flaccid member into her mouth as she can.
20. This time she does the same thing but with an erection.
21. One-way massage:
    a. from the tip down
    b. in the opposite direction
22. retracting and returning the foreskin to its resting position:
    a. on a flaccid member
    b. on an erect one
23. The woman grabs the member with her lips and lets go of it. This is repeated many times in different positions:
    a. with the man lying on his back with an erection
    b. in the same position but this time with no erection
    c. standing up without an erection
24. Retracting the foreskin all the way off the tip:
    a. with a hand on the penis
    b. with a hand on the testicles
25. This massage is very similar to the one described in point 14, but this time the woman grabs the member with her lips. This massage can be performed with the man:
    a. standing up
    b. sitting down
26. The woman places the penis in her mouth and sucks it as if trying to get something out.
27. As the man lies on his back with an erection, she raises his penis to a vertical position or beyond it if possible and massages it orally.

28. The woman is on her back this time with her partner kneeling over her with no or just a partial erection:
    a. the woman performs the massage
    b. the man moves his member in and out of his partner's mouth as she squeezes her lips trying not to let it go
29. The man stands in front of his partner with an erection, and he:
    a. moves his penis around in her mouth without taking it out
    b. takes it out of her mouth after each move
    c. takes it out once in a while
30. The man is standing with no erection in front of his sitting partner. The woman places the flaccid member into her mouth and turns her head to the right until it slips out. Then the action is repeated in the other direction.
31. Rubbing the glans penis against the inner cheek of his partner's mouth:
    a. this can be done by the woman
    b. or the man can also perform this massage himself
32. In this massage the man can either be standing up or lying down. The woman places herself perpendicular to his body and moves her lips along the penis in both directions.
33. The man is on his back with a full erection. The woman pulls the scrotum until the penis assumes the vertical position and then she performs the oral massage.
34. Moving her tongue along the inner side of his member.
35. A frenulum massage done with her tongue through the foreskin.
36. A frenulum massage done with her tongue after retracting the foreskin.
37. She uses her tongue to massage the glans penis and the corona.

38. The woman holds the penis in her mouth and massages it with her tongue.
39. She puts pressure on the penis with her teeth through the foreskin.
40. The woman puts very gentle pressure on the penis after retracting the foreskin.
41. She gently moves the foreskin back and forth with her teeth.
42. One uses her teeth to softly bite the shaft of the penis.
43. She performs an oral massage while massaging the testicles with her hand.
44. The woman massages the shaft of the penis with her hand while simultaneously performing an oral massage.
45. Massaging the scrotum and testes:
    a. with her lips
    b. with her tongue
    c. with her mouth and tongue
    d. while placing one or both testicles in her mouth
    e. stretching the scrotum with her lips

The massage techniques described at the beginning of the chapter (mostly for beginners) can also be used in more advanced and therapeutic massages. They can but do not have to be modified, and just because they are simple to master, they should not be discredited. This is why they are ideal for beginners and useful for everyone.

CHAPTER 12

Intimate Massage Healing

I think everyone is aware of how important to a man is his sex life and his performance in bed. If something does not work as well as expected, his ego suffers. Even if his partner assures him that there is nothing to worry about and everything is all right, it is usually to no avail. Below are some of the most basic problems that guys face and methods he and his partner can share to conquer them.

As I have mentioned a few times before, the method of healing with intimate massage, as well as healing with sex, is based on inducing sexual arousal and keeping it going for an appropriate amount of time. The amount of time is very important because only after prolonged sexual activity (about an hour) does one's body start producing endorphins, which are responsible for good mood and feelings. When enough endorphins are produced, a process of self-healing starts to take place. There is nothing strange about it; it is not a miracle; it is not magic; it is nature. After all, an ancient proverb says, "The doctor dresses the wound and God heals it."

This self-healing process can be channeled to any part of the body. It is not limited to a certain area or to combating just a few problems. Intimate massage can be used to help solving problems of an intimate nature just as well as other health problems that have nothing to do with intimacy. To be more specific—it can be used to help:

- most physical ailments
- emotional problems
- mood issues
- lack of joy of life/depression
- nervous problems/anxiety
- restore inner peace

Although the body and mind may seem like two separate entities, they are actually connected and work closely together. Your psychological state directly affects your physical health and vice versa. So when the brain releases endorphins*, they improve your psychological state, which in turn positively affect the body, helping it heal.

Intimate massage can be a tool to help quitting additions. It will not solve the problem by itself, but it can bring you closer to success when combined with other means. If you have such a problem, convince yourself, for starters, to substitute whatever it is you are addicted to, just once, with an hour of intimate massage. See what it feels like and how it affects your mood, even long after the massage is over. Perhaps experiencing those benefits on yourself can help you come to the decision to change your habits. Intimate massage offers you the opportunity to do just that, but your cooperation is needed to succeed. Massage calms, relaxes, and brings inner peace. Of course, it stimulates the production of large amounts of endorphins. You feel great, and that is the purpose of the massage, but after you leave the therapist's office, what you do for the rest of the day is up to you. To continue feeling great throughout the day, you should make an effort to have an optimistic outlook on life, to be cheerful, to think positively. The effects of stress can discombobulate your whole system. So next time you feel frustrated, stressed, crave a smoke, or have any other negative emotion, indulge in an erotic-intimate massage. Contact with another person is important in those moments, and when the endorphins start to kick in you will feel much better and will be able to take pleasure from life again. When you learn to control your weaknesses with the help of intimate massage—that is a victory.

I want to go over a few health problems, because in order to get rid of them, you must first understand them. Of course it is even better to know how they work to prevent them rather than heal them later.

I will start with men's sexual problems first, as those are relatively easy to cure* with intimate massage. The "therapist" can be his partner or a professional masseuse. Not all men are comfortable with sharing their intimate problems with their partners, and that is when a masseuse comes in handy. It does not have to be a professional; this book can serve as a guide for amateurs who want to learn and practice this type of massage.*

Side note

The work of a massage therapist* (see **"Masseuse"** and **"Intimate massage parlor"**), an intimate massage specialist, should not be compared to the work of a prostitute. A therapist is like a nurse who specializes in massages. If it is acceptable to massage the buttocks, why should it be any different with a penis? Besides, it is much better to heal naturally than to use methods that cause unwanted side effects**(10)**. As you may know, massage regulates circulation, and the better the blood flow the stronger the erection. Circulation also affects sensations in women. It only makes sense to include intimate areas in your massage because of the many benefits it brings.

Lack of sexual appetite

Some middle-aged men whose sexual activity has become lesser than it was earlier in life may experience a decrease in libido. One of the reasons for that is less testosterone in the body. Testosterone is a hormone responsible for regulating the sex drive. Tests to measure the levels of testosterone in the body are available at doctors' offices. It is also a good idea to check your levels of prolactine.*

Another common reason for the loss of sexual appetite in men is due to a neglected relationship. The loss of interest in sex may be caused by a woman's indifference to intimate play or from her desire to dominate the man. In such cases, action has to be taken quickly or the relationship will fall apart.

If a woman shows too much interest in sex (in the man's opinion), it may be perceived as unattractive behavior. A partner who doesn't seem to show any interest is not beneficial either. It is not easy to please a man, isn't it?

Faking an orgasm is never a good idea and can cause a decrease of interest in sexual activity. If a woman fakes an orgasm (and the man does not realize it), the man thinks he is satisfying her needs and does not change anything in his behavior. The woman suffers from not being able to climax and the man thinks everything is fine. The woman's frustration is greater if she has had an orgasm before and knows the pleasure of it.

It is possible to lose interest in sex by revealing too much information about past relationships to each other. Such an approach can cause problems even if a person assures the other that the past does not matter. Even though the assurance may be honest, the truth can still cause pain and aversion to your partner. Partners can become jealous of each other even because of the past . . . which supposedly does not matter. Therefore, it's best to skip over the tales of past erotic adventures and focus on the present.

Erectile dysfunction

There is a prevalent stereotype in our culture that makes a man responsible for his and his partner's satisfaction. Most women may deny this claim, but unfortunately the situation seems helpless when seen through the eyes of a man. Especially young men have a tendency to look at sex as another sport activity, where intimacy equals a series of repeated acrobatics. If you treat sex as yet another task to accomplish, to prove to yourself you are a person of success, you are causing more harm than good because you are blocking your emotions. Their lack or diminished presence can occur for a long period of time, possibly leading to a loss of interest in sex, discouragement with sexual activities, and even depression. Because an erection is a reflection of a man's health, problems with it can suddenly manifest themselves and quickly intensify if left untreated

You may ask yourself, "When should I start worrying?" The truth is, you shouldn't, because that is not going to solve the problem. Instead, you should research the subject to find the cause of the issue. A healthy male should have an erection a few times a night and should also experience "morning wood," an erection occurring in the morning while waking up; of course masturbation should also cause an erection. If that is the case, the possible erection problems have psychological and physical causes, which is actually good news. For example, if you have no problem getting hard during self-stimulation but not around your partner, the problem is likely in your head. Perhaps you are having performance anxiety or "stage fright," or maybe there is a different cause that you have not discovered yet. Erectile dysfunction may be a temporary problem, and the worst thing you can do is tell yourself you will be impotent for the rest of your life.

The frequency of an erection has a lot to do with age. Young men have the greatest ability to get a hard-on. With age the frequency decreases. Young males also experience a stronger, fuller erection because blood fully fills the Corpus Cavernosum**(see Glossary)** penis, while older men usually experience a weaker erection—due to changes in their vascular system.

If you are experiencing problems with your erection, you should consult a physician to determine the cause. If the cause is arteriosclerosis, then on top of medications and massage, a change of lifestyle is often necessary. Each case should be treated individually. Waiting for the problem to go away on its own is usually the worst thing to do.

In order to overcome these problems, a man needs the help of his partner—a loving and understanding woman who can show him needed affection. If he cannot or does not want to count on his partner, a therapist can become a substitute. Therapists cannot assure the love a partner can but they can offer professionalism.

Side note

It is important to remember that manhood is not synonymous with sexual ability, as impotence pill producers would have us believe. They want people to think the only way to be a "real man" is to buy their products. They make it seem as if the only way to get a rock-solid hard-on is to pop a pill.

The antidote to sex problems is intimate massage. However, in order to be effective, the sessions must fulfill the following requirements:

- They must take place in a comfortable, trustful environment.
- The duration of each session must always be taken into account. This is important because the brain starts producing endorphins about an hour after the beginning of sexual stimulation.
- Each massage must be diversified to avoid monotony and a decrease in arousal.
- A massage should be fun.
- Massage should be complemented with a change of lifestyle, if necessary.
- Partners should encourage each other to perform a massage.

Exercise: Genital massage

It is best to do this exercise with your partner, but if you prefer to start out by yourself, it is okay too. The aim of this exercise is to increase blood flow to the penis by gently massaging it, especially at its base, ten to fifteen minutes a day.

The goal here is not to get an erection (although it may very well appear), but to get to know your body's reactions to specific stimuli. Try to repeat this exercise every day, preferably with your partner.

Exercise: Conscious erection

It may strike some of you as odd that not every man can tell if he has an erection when he is excited. This exercise is designed to help those men become aware of their hard-on.

To make it easier, create a scale of hardness of the penis, one being flaccid and ten being rock hard. Before beginning this exercise with your partner, try to revise the scale alone, during a morning erection or self-stimulation. When the time comes to start the exercise, lie on your back with your eyes closed and have your partner start massaging your chest and legs and slowly transition into caressing your genitals, gradually increasing the stimuli. Have your partner gauge your erection on the previously established scale a few times during the massage. Do not treat this exercise as you would a mountain hike: the object isn't to reach level eight, nine, or ten right away but to learn to precisely gauge it without looking at your penis.

Exercise: How to regain what you have lost

Of course I am talking about the ability to regain an erection, after you go limp. Many men have a problem regaining an erection if they lose it in an intimate situation. Losing an erection is not something unusual, it can happen to *anyone*, but getting the erection back might not be easy. This sometimes happens because of the great stress caused by the initial loss of an erection, and even the most pleasurable stimuli may be useless.

The key in solving this problem is relaxation. You need to learn how to achieve this stage. Lie on your back and have your partner start a relaxing massage, going through sensual massage and eventually transitioning into an intimate massage. Finally, an oral massage should be performed until you reach a visible erection. When that happens the stimulation should be paused until you become completely flaccid again (you can help the process along by squeezing your Kegel or holding your breath). Then the steps should be repeated. If you reach a higher level of excitement, that is good, but do not try to force anything. If you are having trouble reaching an erection while lying down, try kneeling while your partner lies down. That way you will get better circulation to your member.

When your partner or your doctor cannot solve your problem, the medication Viagra can be helpful. Within thirty minutes of taking it, a man is ready for intercourse and the erection can last as long as four hours. You should not decide to take it on your own; always consult a physician first because a doctor is able to find the cause of the dysfunction and may decide that another course of action should be taken. If the cause of erectile dysfunction is from a serious ailment, even Viagra will not be able to help. If the cause is lack of blood reaching the penis, then sex-enhancing drugs may be helpful.

Viagra is a good medication, but there are other ways of combating erectile dysfunction. Scientists have discovered that oils are rich in a sex hormone called prostaglandins. Walnut oil, flax oil, and wheat sprout oil work the best. Sunflower oil is good too. Pure potency with no side effects, though you should always use as directed.

Side note

If you want to help your man overcome his erectile dysfunction, you must forget about showing any anger or dissatisfaction caused by unfulfilled desires. If you cannot do that, do not attempt the "therapy" so you do not unintentionally make things worse. Such a procedure requires time and patience—and above all, a cheerful disposition. During the "therapy", both partners rediscover each other and their own bodies and desires by arousing one another.

When attempting to treat impotence at home, a few rules must be followed. Intercourse is not allowed for six weeks so that the man is not, in any way, responsible for achieving an orgasm. He is only to caress and be caressed—so that he does not have to stress out about holding back an orgasm and dissatisfying his partner in case he fails to do so.

Premature ejaculation: What does it really mean?

There is no definition that sets an ideal or even correct time for the duration of intercourse. However, a general classification of premature ejaculation is a climax reached before penetration, shortly after the beginning of intercourse, or simply earlier than the man would like. Basically it is when he has no control over how fast he ejaculates.

It is generally considered that premature ejaculation primarily affects young men who are just starting to have sex. In reality, it is the most common sexual disorder(11) and can happen to anyone. A short duration of intercourse is normal at the beginning of a sex journey or after a long interval of no sex. However, it can become a source of frustration in any other case. If you think you do not have adequate control of your ejaculation, the exercises on the following pages may prove to be helpful.

What are the causes?

Usually the lack of or limited control of the Kegel muscle causes premature ejaculation (more on the Kegel muscle in Chapter 4). The problem stems from the brain and from the fear of poor performance intensified by, for example, a new partner. To overcome the problem, one has to learn to control the Kegel muscle, be relaxed in bed, and be aware of experiencing the sensations occurring at the moment. Concentrating on something else other than what one is doing at the time is not good.

First, remember that sex is not a sport. The goal is not to have the best finishing time or to beat the other "contestants." Depending on the mood and other circumstances you may want a "quickie" or may desire a long, intimate evening together. There is no point in adapting to any norms. However, if you notice that there might be a problem, it is best if your partner is there to help you solve it. That way you will spend time together working on it.

It is not always possible though, as not everyone has a permanent partner. This is when intimate massage parlors can be of help. They provide qualified professionals with experience and the ability to create the right atmosphere, which enables a man to feel no stress. Besides, not every partner can do a massage, due to, for example, no desire to perform it.

If your partner wants to help, that's great. If not, you should think about seeing a masseuse. You may be asking yourself if you should tell your partner about it. There is no right answer, it depends on many factors, but it may be responsible to ask your partner's opinion on the subject before making a decision.

Side note

Another reason for premature ejaculation may be too much sexual tension. Just an uneasy thought that the intercourse is going to be a failure may in fact make it one. Nervousness can lead to an unwanted climax. In addition, focusing too much on not climaxing can have a negative effect. In such circumstances, failure is all but guaranteed. Great advice regarding such a problem would be to tell the man to stop focusing on those thoughts, but this advice is often impossible to achieve. It works well in theory, but in reality it is practically almost impossible to make it work. It may work for a few if they know some sort of secret technique of control, such as breathing methods.

But what about the majority of men who experience premature ejaculation? How can they overcome their problem? Well, a good way is to turn their attention away from intercourse to delay the orgasm. The best method for achieving that is intimate massage, performed in a relaxed, stress-free setting, during which the masseuse switches up the techniques in order to avoid too-early orgasm. And if it does happen, so what? Nobody is disappointed, nobody feels embarrassed. A masseuse is an understanding person who is familiar with these types of problems, and there is no room for embarrassment.

Sometimes an ejaculation that occurs before a woman's orgasm may be caused by the woman's inability to reach a climax, or her slower reactions to sexual stimulation in comparison to her partner's. Another reason may be a woman's hyperactivity during intercourse. For instance, if she makes unexpected movements, they may cause too much excitement and lead to an orgasm. So not every sexual misfortune is caused by serious physical or psychological issues.

Treatment

Start with Kegel exercises described in Chapter 4. When you feel comfortable, move on to working with your partner. Begin with very simple exercises and gradually gain new ground to eventually feel more in control.

Keep in mind that the following exercises work only if you do not pressure yourself into gaining an erection.

The spring exercise:

1. Lie on your back and ask your partner to make you fully erect. Next, she brings your penis to a vertical position and then lets it go. Now you need to contract your Kegel. The point is to squeeze your Kegel hard enough to stop your member from hitting your belly. Repeat this many times. It can also be done sideways when lying down or standing up. The spring can be performed using a hand or mouth to raise the penis to a vertical position.
2. To make it more interesting, instead of raising the penis directly, gently pull the scrotum to achieve the same result. This method makes the treatment seems more like fun, and that is the whole point.
3. Using lips, you can be sure that your partner will be even more willing to participate in the treatment.
4. When your partner is flaccid, grab his penis and gently squeeze it. Keep a tight grip on it so that you can feel the contracting and relaxing of the Kegel. Stretch the member

forward up or to the sides if it helps you feel it. Ask your man to squeeze his Kegel as you count the reps. Have him do three sets of twenty; it's really worth it.

Exercise: An orgasm with a contracted Kegel

Your Kegel muscle can help you gauge your arousal like a barometer on a scale of one to ten (one being flaccid and ten being an orgasm). Contracting your Kegel once will bring you down a level. Try this by yourself first and then involve your partner.

Start playing with yourself and continue until you climax. During the masturbation, squeeze your Kegel in different ways: one strong squeeze, two medium contractions, a few quick ones, etc., to figure out which method works best. Remember that squeezing it too hard before reaching a full erection may cause it to go flaccid for a moment. Learn to maneuver this muscle (like the gears of a manual transmission; downshift or put it in reverse to postpone the climax).

When you master the ability of contracting and relaxing your Kegel, start exercising with your partner. Take it slowly at first, with gentle petting of the genitals. When you feel that you have reached a high level of arousal on the one to ten scale and are close to the culmination point, squeeze the Kegel using the method you have discovered earlier that works best for you. Contract and release it a few times, allowing yourself to take a deep breath between each squeeze. When you are really close to an orgasm, try to come down of one level on the aforementioned scale.

Repeat this exercise a few more times. As progress is made, your partner can use more intense stimuli. Your partner and her attitude play an important role in the process. It is very good if you can count on her patience and understanding. Unfortunately, some women wrongly assume that a premature ejaculation is nothing but a man's selfishness. They think that it happens because he only cares about his own satisfaction. If you do experience an early climax, just wait a moment and start over.

Some men who suffer from sexual disorders just get better intrinsically. It is not a miracle. Here are some of the possible reasons:

- Cutting out a stressful factor. For example, a man who suffers from premature ejaculation and focuses on his problem fearing his woman's dissatisfaction can find a partner who has clitoral orgasms and does not care how long the sex lasts.
- Living a healthier lifestyle, which is not necessarily associated with having an affect on sex. For instance, a man with an erectile dysfunction starts using the car less, changes his diet, quits smoking, etc.
- Elimination of an unknown ailment causing the problem; for example, addressing a circulation problem or treating high blood pressure.
- Discontinuing the use of some medication. Only a handful of doctors inform their patients of the side effects of some prescription drugs on men's and woman's sex lives. Most of the drugs that have a negative effect on intimacy are sedatives and painkillers, blood pressure meds, ulcer drugs, appetite suppressants, migraine medicine, and many over-the-counter drugs (for example, allergy meds or rhinitis drugs). All those can cause erectile problems.

I am convinced that treatment of ejaculation problems, as well as other sexual disorders should start with intimate massage. Men who suffer from these problems can learn to control their arousal to the point right before the involuntary climax. The technique of controlling your arousal is helpful for those men who climax so fast that neither they nor their partners get any satisfaction. Give these exercises a try and you will see how effective they can be.

Penis desensitizing massage: to slow down an orgasm

1. Lie on your back. Your partner gives you an intimate massage without any lubrication. Close your eyes and focus on the sensations. When an orgasm is approaching, ask your partner to take a quick break until your arousal decreases a bit. Keep repeating this exercise until you can successfully go on for fifteen minutes without stopping, and then proceed to the next one.

2. Do the same as described in the previous exercise, but this time use lube. Lubrication makes a big difference, so it will be much harder to control an orgasm. When a climax is near, ask your partner to stop until you feel less aroused.

3. Lube up both your hands and alternate sliding them down his penis from the tip down the shaft to the base. First use one hand and then the other in a constant motion for a few minutes. This is very exciting because it feels different than regular petting. It can be done in any position. Depending on the way you like it, your partner can apply more or less pressure. This method is quite helpful with erectile issues.

4. Massage your partner's penis with or without lube. When reaching climax, instead of her taking her hand away, squeeze it for fifteen to thirty seconds. This will stop the

orgasm and reduce the arousal. Then the massage can be continued. If the penis goes flaccid, ask your partner to grab it at the base with her thumb and index finger. Then have her jerk it up and down for a few minutes (in one-to two-second intervals). This should be repeated many times before an ejaculation is allowed.

5. Your woman lubes up the tip of your penis (if you are uncircumcised, retract the foreskin), and massages it. It is a highly sensitive area, and this exercise may be quite exciting. In order to see results, this should be done regularly. At first an orgasm can be quick, but with time there will be visible progress.

6. Lie on your back and have your partner sit between your legs facing you. Using lubrication, she massages the tip of the penis. Your partner should be watching your reactions and should stop the massage when she notices pre-cum. After waiting a moment, the massage should be continued—but ejaculation should not be allowed just yet. Sometimes a good method of preventing an orgasm is to squeeze the penis a few times below the tip. The squeeze should be hard but not painful. This exercise should be performed for thirty minutes daily, for about two weeks. After that, it should be continued for a year, at first in weekly and then monthly intervals. Therapists often use this method.

7. You and your partner should determine how long it takes you to regenerate after ejaculation. When you figure it out, have your partner stimulate you until you climax. Wait until you can go again and then have sex. If the experiment works, next time wait longer before you have sex after the initial orgasm. Each time extend the waiting period a little to bring about more control.

Methods of preventing an ejaculation during sex:

1. The first method involves squeezing the penis for about three seconds. It should be done below the tip. It cannot be too hard, so it does not hurt and the erection does not go away.
2. Squeezing and gently pulling down the scrotum at the base of the member for ten to thirty seconds also prevents an orgasm. Be careful not to squeeze the testicles themselves but in a spot a little above them where the scrotum meets the penis.
3. Pressing the "holy spot"—the place between the anus and the scrotum—is a method known in China since antiquity. Applying pressure to that spot for ten to thirty seconds reverses the course of the ejaculation energy. The pressure should be gentle yet firm and applied with two fingers. Over time, the pressure should gradually decrease.
4. When you feel you are near a climax, stop all friction, and after a few moments you can go back to doing it. It is a convenient method because you do not even have to take your penis out of her vagina.

Some exercises to prevent an unwanted orgasm:

In order for the methods described above to work correctly, you have to practice them with your partner. They require some experience, though. There are moments when you cannot spend a few seconds looking for the right spot, and you have to know where it is or the exercise is over. So, practice the following:

- Squeezing the penis—as described in point 1) above.
- The proper squeezing and pulling of the scrotum—see point 2).

- Applying pressure to the "holy spot"—refer to point 3).
- Refer to point 4) above for information on how to use friction (and when to stop using it) but with the use of hands instead of a vagina.

This exercise can also be done using lips, but using hands might have more control over the arousal of your partner because of the different levels of pressure that can be applied with the fingers. When executed correctly, this method can quickly bring about positive changes.

Additional methods for delaying an orgasm:

- A hot bath, taken right before intercourse, usually delays many reactions, extending the duration of the sexual interaction.
- A man can use the Kegel exercises. It is best to do fewer of them but more often. An efficient love muscle ensures a strong erection and also increases the power and prolongs the duration of the orgasm. A man who exercises his Kegel muscle is able to contract it at the first sign of an orgasm and hold it for a while to prevent ejaculation.
- Many breathing techniques stem directly from Tantra. Advanced yogis are able to delay or stop an ejaculation altogether just by controlling their breathing. As a person nears an orgasm their breathing rate increases, until a climax is reached. That process can be reversed by concentrating on slow, deep breaths. If an orgasm is very near, both partners should remain absolutely motionless.

Testing the effectiveness of impotence drugs(12)

The market is full of impotence pharmaceuticals, which many men use with varied results. Instead of blindly taking those medications, there is an easy way to check whether they work.

The purpose of testing different drugs is to check their effectiveness in a particular area. There is no point in taking them if there is no guarantee that they are going to work. So test your drugs.

First thing to do is to check the sexual potency of a man. The test should include:

1. Checking your partner's reaction to different stimuli:
    a. An erotic massage (the massage of the chest, abdomen and thighs)
    b. Holding a hand on the testicles without any stimulation
    c. A testicle massage
    d. Holding the penis without making any movements
    e. A massage of the penis
    f. A testicle massage with his penis in your mouth but no other oral stimulation
    g. An oral massage without the use of hands
    h. An oral massage with the use of your hands
2. Checking the duration of:
    a. The stimulation before an erection is apparent
    b. An erection when stimulation has been stopped
    c. An erection with stimulation
3. Checking the time it takes to regain an erection after an ejaculation. After completing the series of test, choose some and repeat the exam after taking the medication. The tests should be repeated a few times:

- Thirty minutes after taking the drug
- Sixty minutes after taking it
- Ninety minutes after its ingestion
- Three hours after the medication has been taken
- Twenty-four hours after the ingestion of the medicine
- Forty-eight hours after the drug has entered the body

The results of each test should be written down and analyzed to answer the following questions:

1. Does the drug work? If you see a difference in the results of the tests done before and after taking the drug (in the patient's favor, of course), it means it works.
2. If it works, how effective is it? You will be able to tell by comparing the results of the tests done before taking the medication to those performed after. The bigger the difference in the results, the more effective the drug.
3. How long does it take for the medication to start working? Compare the results of the tests from before and after taking the drug. Pay close attention to the time after the ingestion of the drug, during which the results are the best. This information will let you know not only when the medication starts working but also when its efficacy peaks.
4. How long do the effects of the medicine last? When the test results start exhibiting a downward trend, it is an infallible sign that the end is near (the end of the effectiveness of the drug that is). For example, when the results start being to the patient's disadvantage three hours after ingesting the drug, additional testing can be performed in two- to three-hour increments in order to find out when its effects completely wear off.

Side note

Higher levels of testosterone can have an effect on lowering cholesterol levels. When no medication is working, one should try those techniques of intimate massage that affect the increase of testosterone concentration in the body.

Check the results of cholesterol after two or three months of using the proper massage. It makes sense only for people with high cholesterol problems.

CHAPTER 13

The Anatomy of Female Bliss

Women's excitement is not as obvious as men's because of the anatomical differences between the two genders. A woman does not necessarily have to be aware of her arousal. So many different processes occur at the same time that it might be difficult to notice visible changes.

A woman's equivalent of a penis is the clitoris. When a female is excited, blood rushes to the clit, causing an erection. Both inner and outer labia look different when excited. They swell up, and the inner lips' color intensifies. The walls of the vagina start secreting mucus, and the muscles that support the uterus tighten up, while the vagina opens up.

The matter of a female orgasm has been widely debated. There used to be many supporters of the theory that climaxing was solely men's domain. Such an idea seems absurd today, when female sexuality is no longer mysterious and inscrutable.

According to Freud, there are two types of female orgasms: clitoral and vaginal, the latter being the "better" of the two. There was another popular theory that stated female orgasms could only be clitoral. However, that theory was dismissed with the discovery of the G-spot (named after Dr. Ernest Grafenberg), which is located on the front wall of the vagina about two inches from its entrance. Since only some women experience the pleasure from stimulating this area, there are skeptics of the G-spot. It has been observed that an orgasm caused by the stimulation of the G-spot is accompanied by a release of a fluid, an equivalent of a male ejaculation. The composition of this fluid is similar to that of semen.

Aside from those described above, there are other areas on the female body that can cause an orgasm. One such place is the urethra. There are woman who climax when their cervix is stimulated. The vaginal cavity, which is located behind the cervix and is usually not accessible, opens up during a time of strong arousal, also becoming a source of pleasure. Caressing the breasts and nipples is obviously part of a bedroom repertoire, though usually more as an appetizer than a main course. However, there are women who are able to have an orgasm just by having their nipples and areolas sucked and rubbed. As incredible as it sounds, it is possible to have an orgasm with just the use of a brain. A fantasy or dream can cause a powerful physical reaction. After waking from such dream, a woman feels as if she actually just had incredible sex. Apart from that, a woman's physiology also indicates that fact.

What goes on in the body during an orgasm? A female orgasm is much more subtle than a male climax, and that is why it is easier to fake. One may be surprised to find that some women have never experienced an orgasm. Many of those women do not admit it to their partners in order not to hurt them, but by lying, they are further reducing their chances of having an orgasm. During an orgasm, blood pressure increases, the heart starts beating rapidly, and breathing increases. Involuntary muscle contractions start at the extremities and travel to the Kegel muscle. The abdomen may start shivering vigorously, and the body feels warm all over. This built-up energy is finally released, leaving the woman feeling ecstatic and satisfied. It is quite a common description, but in reality, the intensity of an orgasm will vary. The same person can experience a climax that is just pleasant one time but feels like an incredible explosion another time.

What if a woman cannot get satisfaction? The first step is to home in on the cause of the problem. There are usually two possibilities: a lack of harmony between partners, or something in the psyche of the woman. If a man pays attention only to himself and his needs, always taking the same (usually the least time-consuming) approach, then it is definitely an obstacle for his partner and her orgasm.

In reality, when it comes to caring couples, only in rare cases does the man put his needs over his partner's. Actually, it is usually the other way around; it is the man's priority to make sure his woman is satisfied. Needless to say, observing a woman having an orgasm is a powerful stimulus. As I have mentioned before, oftentimes it is the woman's fault by not saying anything to her partner about the problem because she does not want to hurt him. A man who is convinced that he is a great lover is not necessarily going to want to experiment or change techniques. The reason for this problem is a lack of communication and a superficial closeness in the bedroom, a place where deep and basic bonds are built and maintained. It is never too late to suggest some new ideas to your partner; so, do not be afraid to start an honest conversation about your needs. What except for an illusion do you have to lose?

Oftentimes the source of the lack of sexual satisfaction lies in a woman's psyche. There are many possible causes of such a problem, but they often start in childhood years. For example, a prude upbringing can be a reason. Problems can stem from being taught at an early age that physicality and everything connected to it is a "sin" and sexual intercourse is to be used only for procreation. Lack of fulfillment in an adult can also be caused by molestation or rape experienced at a young age. The trauma caused by such an event acts as a block, which prevents a person from enjoying sex, and the help of a mental health professional is often necessary.

Other times the problems with satisfaction can be caused by being too self-conscious about our bodies. Of course we can blame the media for promoting certain standards, but women must remember that the bedroom is not a catwalk and that different criteria of attractiveness apply there. It is not perfect measurements that make a happy lover but knowing one's body and opening up to a partner with all the senses. Besides, men tend to be much more liberal than magazines when it comes to female beauty, and they usually do not prefer just one specific type of woman.

Yet another cause of dissatisfaction is the inner necessity of having an orgasm, often additionally fueled by a man who asks his partner every time whether she's had one. That takes all the pleasure out of sex, making it seem like a test of sorts, causing stress.

The stress can also come from outside factors. Many women cannot turn off their thoughts and focus on being close with their partners. Too many persistent thoughts about everyday problems prevent them from concentrating on the "here and now." Instead of passion, which is a source of our energy, we get another chore to cross off the daily to-do list. Fortunately, this problem can be also solved if both people are willing to work on it. The massage techniques described later in the book can help you *carpe diem* (seize the day) in the bedroom on a daily basis.

Earlier in the book I mentioned the importance of knowing one's body in order to have a successful love life. It means that masturbation is a necessary practice if a person really wants to know his or her needs. It should not be treated as a consolation prize when a partner is not around but a rightful part of everyone's intimacy. Isn't it great when everything is literally in your hands?

CHAPTER 14

Arousal, Desire, and Orgasm

Sexual problems that affect women are usually different from those that affect men. Men's sexual problems usually manifest as physical issues, such as erectile dysfunction or problems with ejaculation, while women's problems tend to be psychological in nature. Those problems include a decrease in libido and difficulties with getting aroused. Women can also experience physical issues such as pain during intercourse, but that can be a symptom of psychological problems.

Many people consider arousal and desire to be the same thing. In reality those are two very different things. Arousal is created by the release of hormones, while desire is something much more complicated. There are many different factors that, when compiled together, form libido, including mood and how people get along with each other. It is possible to be aroused without feeling any desire and still be able to have sex. A decrease in libido can often be attributed to some form of depression or trauma, or to age, of course. Resolving medical issues should start with a visit to a doctor who specializes in those kinds of problems.

A few words about problems with arousal. Many women notice that their vaginas are not wet enough during intimate encounters. Most of the time it does not have anything to do with a lack of desire, which can be present even if there is little or no arousal. If that happens, do not waste time worrying about it, just use a lubricant and focus on your feelings. Also, try not to feel frustrated because it takes longer to become aroused. Oftentimes men make the mistake of being impatient and rushing through, or completely skipping foreplay to get to the intercourse. If that is the case, take the initiative to show your partner what you really want.

Exercise: using a vibrator for the first time

Take it easy at the beginning. You have to get used to the new toy and its applications. Lie on your back and gently caress your genitals with the vibrator. When you feel ready, insert it into your vagina, contract, and then relax your Kegel muscle, stimulating your clitoris at the same time. Intuition should guide you to an orgasm. When you feel you are about to climax, slide the vibrator into your vagina.

Exercise: having a "threesome"

I do not mean inviting a third person into your bedroom; instead, try incorporating a vibrator into your intimate games to increase your pleasure.

Lie on your back and have your partner start stimulating your genitals with his hands or mouth. Position your legs in a way that will allow your partner to easily kneel between them and use the vibrator to massage your intimate area. He should start out slowly, gradually increasing the speed. Next have him alternate the stimulation of the clitoris with the stimulation of the Kegel muscles. To stimulate the Kegel, use only the tip of the toy, sliding it in and out of the vagina. After a few minutes, ask him to put the vibrator deeper inside and thrust it in and out a few times. This should further stimulate the Kegel. If it starts to shiver and contract, it means you are close to climaxing.

Exercise: a fast orgasm

The purpose of this exercise is to prove that it does not have to take long to reach an orgasm. It is good news for you as well as your man because men often feel insecurities concerning this issue.

Have your partner lie on his back and please him orally. When he is fully erect, squat over him and rub your clitoris and vaginal lips on his member, but do not allow penetration. After a while, if the erection weakens, return to stimulating it with your mouth. You can also try the "69 position," which is exciting for both. Do not forget to go back to rubbing your genitals with your partner's penis. When you feel you are close to climaxing, take a deep breath and insert the penis into your vagina as you squeeze your Kegel muscle. Satisfaction is guaranteed.

CHAPTER 15

Breast Massage

Breast massage is used for a few different reasons:

- to arouse a woman during foreplay and intercourse
- to relax her
- to make the breasts more firm
- to make them more sensitive

Various breast massage positions:

- on her back
- prone, with her torso slightly elevated
- sitting up straight
- sitting, slightly leaning forward (like on a bike), the breasts are in a different position compared to when sitting up straight
- on all fours

The masseur's positions during a breast massage:

- Straddling the woman who is lying on her back. Remember to use your heels to support your body weight. You can also sit beside or behind her.
- While your partner is sitting, sit or stand behind her. Place a mirror in front of you to make it more interesting.
- When your partner is lying on her belly leaning on her elbows, sit in front, facing her. This arrangement provides an interesting experience for both of you.
- Sit next to your partner with one arm around her and use your other hand to massage her breasts.
- Sit behind your woman, and as you caress her breasts, whisper in her ear or kiss her neck.
- Have your partner lie down on your thighs as you are sitting up. This position is usually used in really close relationships.

You can perform a breast massage using:

- Your hands. Always start gently touching the areas around the breasts. Massage the sides of her torso, her belly, and the space between the breasts. When you reach her breasts use concentric movements starting from the outside toward the nipples.
- Your lips and tongue. Those are exciting tools of the trade that excite both the giver and the receiver of the massage.
- A stream of water. Experimenting with water can be an unforgettable experience that has additional benefits: cleansing and firming/toning the skin.
- Various accessories, such as handheld massage instruments, vibrators (which can be turned on or off), peacock feathers, fringes, or silk.

- Your penis. You can do the massage or let her use your penis to rub her breasts and nipples. A woman's imagination may work wonders.

Very gentle touching or tickling the breasts makes them sensitive to touch. This is why some women begin to experience pleasure from breast stimulation only after some time. You can also massage through a delicate material, such as silk or velvet.

You can also lube your hands with massage oil or spread talcum powder on your partner's body. It is worth trying new methods of which some you will like and others you will not, it all depends on personal preferences and your sensitivity to different stimuli. Most often a massage is done with little or no lubrication, but it is fun to experiment. I especially recommend a breast massage performed with really oily hands. The breasts just slide through the fingers and it feels really good for both.

Different ways of massaging the breasts:

1. Alternate circular and sliding motions on the sides of the breasts.
2. Using the fingers of hands, massage the top and sides of the breasts, omitting the nipples. This works especially well if you sit behind your partner.
3. Massage the bottom of the breasts with your thumbs.
4. Use your thumbs to gently press in the nipples and massage them in a circular motion.
5. Pull the nipples.
6. Twist the nipples.
7. Rub the space between her nipples, "accidentally" touching them.
8. Suck the nipples.

9. Pull the nipples with your lips.
10. Lick them.
11. Simultaneously massage both breasts using your fingers, starting on the outside and moving in towards the nipples.
12. Gently squeeze one breast with one hand.
13. Gently pull one breasts with a hand.
14. Gently alternate squeezing and pulling one breast with one hand.
15. Repeat points 12, 13, and 14 but with the other breast.
16. Do the same as above but to both breasts at the same time now.
17. Now, massage one breast with both hands and then repeat with the other breast.
18. Put a hand on one of her breasts and massage the other one with your other hand. Then switch it up.
19. Put one hand on one breast while using your other hand to massage the other breast from the outside in, with a clockwise motion.
20. Do the same as the point above, but using a counterclockwise motion.
21. Repeat the past few steps but for both breasts simultaneously.
22. Using your fingers, massage each part of one breast with small circular movements while keeping the other breast covered with your other hand. Keep alternating breasts until both have been fully massaged.
23. Slide your hands across the breasts from side to side
24. Slide your hands up and down the breasts.
25. Squeeze the breasts together.
26. Pull the breasts apart.
27. When the woman is sitting or standing, raise the breasts with your hands and let them drop.

28. While the woman is sitting down stretch the breasts up and down.
29. Stimulate the breasts with your tongue.
30. Using your fingers, outline the breasts in a "figure 8" motion.
31. Gently squeeze the breasts.
32. Put your hands on her breasts, gently squeeze and move them in a circular motion.
33. Slide your hands up and down her body from her neck to belly no omitting her breasts.
34. Place your hands on the breasts with your fingers spread wide apart on their sides and move them in towards the nipples.
35. Put some massage oil on the breasts and slowly start massaging them in a circular motion from the outside in. When you get to the nipples, they should already be erected and hard. It is the most commonly recommended and used method by specialists.

Breast exam

From time to time each woman should examine her breasts on her own. Of course, it would be better her man to do it instead but at first she needs to learn it herself. So, let's start.

- Stand in front of a mirror. Visually examine your breasts with your arms at your sides, then with your hands on your hips, and then with your arms raised over your head. Changing the position of your arms will allow you to notice any changes in the shape of your breasts or any changes of the skin. Observe if the skin gets wrinkly anywhere or if it pulls in any spot.
- Squeeze your nipple and observe if any liquid is secreted.

- While standing up, raise one arm and check the breast with your palm, moving it in a circular motion from the outside in.
- Lie on your back, put your left hand under your head, and place a pillow under your left arm. Using your right hand, examine your left breast. Then, do the same with the right breast, switching your position accordingly.
- While lying down, place your left arm parallel to your body and using your right hand check the outer part of your left breast. Do the same thing on the other side of your body. Possible problems can usually be located between the armpit and the bottom of the ribs.
- A bath can also be a good time for an exam. When touching a soapy breast, gently press your fingers toward your ribs. Even if the smallest bump is there, you should be able to detect it.

CHAPTER 16

The Joy of Intimate Massage

Intimate massage can be performed with:

- hands
- finger or multiple fingers
- lips
- tongue
- penis (both hard and flaccid)
- accessories (vibrators, dildos, Ben-Wa balls, beads, a small brush or brushes, or a shaving brush—it is worth a try)

Intimate massage for women

Satisfaction with one's sex life determines the success of a relationship. This means that everyone should work on themselves and strive to understand their partner's and their own needs and then fulfill them as much as possible.

Physical contact should ideally take place in an emotional relationship. The act of sexual intercourse should be a complement of a relationship between two people who love each other. It should not happen before a strong emotional bond is established between the partners. This is especially true for women, who need more love and affection. When a woman feels needed and loved, she is more likely to experience full sexual satisfaction, and her erotic experiences tend to be much deeper compared to a woman who is in a physical relationship and does not feel loved. Intimate massage also has an impact on a woman's sexual psyche development. This contact between partners has to take place with a certain level of emotional involvement. Only then the woman will experience the desired satisfaction. It is important to have a mutual understanding and to know your partner's needs and desires.

Different types of massages, frequent intercourse, and exercises with a vibrator increase the sensitivity of a woman's intimate parts. Constant stimulation causes a growth of a sexual appetite. A woman must accept herself as she is. No one is perfect, but everyone is attractive and beautiful in their own way. It is important to realize this simple truth.

To fully enjoy intimate moments, one must first change his or (especially) her attitude toward his or her body and nudity. Try doing mental exercises that focus on a positive attitude toward sexual intercourse. Eliminate all words from your vocabulary that have a negative connotation with sex, such as "dirty" and "obscene." Think of it as something beautiful, good, and soothing; after all, it is sharing yourself with your loved one.

Self-massage

Intimate massage should cause pleasure and arousal. However, an orgasm is not the goal. Sometimes it is best to start with a self-massage. By *self-massage* I do not mean masturbation, but

I mean to find out what kind of touch you like the most, what you find pleasurable. If you do this with the right attitude, you will discover that touching yourself brings about a feeling of well being, and that is not selfish at all.

When observing a masturbating women, researchers concluded(13) that there is a variety of techniques that cause arousal in women. Furthermore, they discovered that each woman pleasures herself in a different, unique way. Most frequently they stimulated the whole genital area, which affected the clitoris, regardless of any direct contact with it. So, only *you* can discover how to stimulate your intimate areas in the best way.

Sample exercises

Find yourself a quiet place where you will not be interrupted. Sit or lie down naked in a position most comfortable for you. Remember that touching is not synonymous with masturbating. The purpose of this exercise is to find different, pleasing sensations, and not to reach an orgasm.

Pour a little baby oil or some other moisturizer on your fingers and slowly start touching your inner thighs and labia. If any part of your body seems tense, try to loosen it up. You can limit yourself to touching only the external genitals or you can caress your vagina as well. Just do what causes you pleasure and joy. Concentrate on your touch. Focus on touching your genitals, and if your thoughts start to drift, bring them back to that point.

Try different methods of touching. Caress yourself just as your partner normally would and then switch it up to something different. Pet your inner and outer lips, your clitoris and vaginal opening. Treat all body parts equally, spending the same amount of time on each one. Relax and even out your breathing. Focus on your body and on the changes it undergoes, when touching its different parts. Monitor the changes in skin temperature and surface texture. It is fine if you feel aroused, but remember that it is not the goal at this time. Your goal is to experience pleasure in order to get to know your body. Caress your body slowly and gently to feel sensual delight and joy. Do this for fifteen minutes.

Sit in front of a mirror and spread your legs wide to see yourself from your man's perspective. Spread your outer lips, if they have not done so by themselves already, and then spread your inner labia. Gently rub your clit—and figure out what kind of massage you like the most. Think how you will show your partner how to do the same thing just as openly as at this moment, in full light, without hiding anything. By doing this you will achieve two goals: you will show your partner a better way of arousing you; and you will show him one of the most important visual stimuli, which is your widely spread vagina being stimulated by your finger.

Massage performed by your partner

1. Lie comfortably on the floor or couch and slightly spread your legs. Put your hands alongside your body or under your head. Your partner should start caressing your body using a little bit of talc. When he gets to your genitals, he should use a lot of lube to slowly move his fingers on the outer and inner lips, and the clitoris. Concentrate on his every move. Your man should also focus on his actions. When he slowly inserts a finger into your vagina, he feels its warmth and texture and the muscles surrounding it. During this exercise, your partner can lie between your

legs and not only feel but see what he is doing. He should try to get to know every inch of your skin. If he feels the petting has become automatic, he should slow down and focus on his actions.

2. Another method that drives women crazy is "the hitchhiker." To perform this, you must access your woman from behind with your thumb. When you put your thumb into her vagina from the back, bend it, and the fingertip should land on the G-spot, or in its vicinity. Use your thumb to gently massage that area, which is sure to arouse your partner, and leave her begging for more every time.

3. Have your woman lie on her back on a bed or floor and relax. Slowly start massaging her intimate area with your tongue. When she is somewhat warmed up, insert your middle finger into her vagina without stopping the oral stimulation. Then move your finger up so that it rests on her clitoris. Next, firmly push the clitoris up with your finger and begin licking and sucking it. Simultaneously place your free hand on your partner's belly right above the pubic bone, and while gently pressing, make circular movements.

4. When your woman lies on her back, place her right leg on your shoulder, hence gaining easy access to her pubic mound. Gently and tenderly part your partner's labia, exposing the clitoris, which looks like a butterfly in this position. Brush the clitoris with your tongue and suck on it from time to time, while slowly and gently spreading and squeezing the labia with your index finger and thumb, which should look like a butterfly flapping its wings. By working out a suitable rhythm, the vulva will also get massaged. In order to increase the pleasure, use the thumb of your other hand to slide it in and out of the vagina.

5. Playing with the penis also brings some benefits and a lot of satisfaction. Grab your flaccid or erect penis and move it along the vaginal opening starting at the bottom of the vagina toward the clitoris. Then do it in the opposite direction. This kind of massage not only stimulates your partner, who may or may not have problems with reaching an orgasm, but also arouses you, leading to an ejaculation.

6. Another version of a massage with the penis: sit on the floor with your legs wide apart and your woman kneeling in front of you, facing you. Place the tip of your penis in the vaginal opening, but do not put it all the way in. Instead, use your hand to move your penis around that area. It is a great foreplay, after which intercourse can take place. When both of you feel strong arousal, pull your partner toward you to fully penetrate her.

When your partner is performing a massage, close your eyes and concentrate on what he is doing. Breathe calmly and relax completely. Try to absorb his touch the best way you can. Feel the physical contact and try to forget about reality. If you feel something that you really like, tell your partner about it. He, in turn, should not only listen to your remarks, but also put them into practice. A lot depends on the man and his affection, which is often just as arousing as a sophisticated caress. When dealing with a young lover, who has not had many sexual experiences, a man must act with a lot of skill and patience. Gentle touching is important and a lot of time should be spent on soft kisses, caressing the breasts, hips and buttocks. She has to get used to the fact that those areas can be touched by another person (preferably a trustful and loving one). At the same time, it will be a good opportunity for her body to become more sensitive.

A woman's pleasure increases slowly and the goal is to make her fully enjoy herself. That is why it is important to stimulate her regularly and rhythmically. Those stimuli, which seem very gentle at first, start getting perceived as more distinct and stronger with time, as the arousal increases. The same touch, the same sensation, which at first might have seemed irksome becomes greatly pleasing and arousing.

Intimate massage is really helpful for women who have difficulty climaxing. If a man cannot get his partner adequately aroused, he should perform an intimate massage preceded by a relaxing and erotic massage. Getting her to relax, followed by a delicate arousal, can transform into stronger sensations, which can lead to an orgasm.

Some benefits of erotic and intimate massages:

1. Awakening sexual sensitivity.
2. Making the breasts more firm.
3. Making the breasts more sensitive to touch (young women oftentimes do not feel any pleasure from having their breasts caressed).
4. Improving the quality of the orgasm—a weak orgasm can become more intense.
5. A greater frequency of climaxing.
6. A stronger sensation of pleasure during sex, through the stimulation of the G-spot during the massage.
7. Eliminating the problem of a loose vagina through the use of the Kegel exercises.

A few more tips on how to perform an intimate massage on a woman:

1. Put your hand on the woman's genitals and make circular movements with it.
2. Do the same thing as described above, but this time insert your fingers into the vagina.
3. Do the same as above, but instead of keeping your fingers in the vagina, slide them in and out.
4. Move your fingers in a circular motion on the woman's clitoris.
5. Spread the vaginal lips.
6. Spread the vaginal lips apart and push them together while rubbing them against each other.
7. Rub your finger between the labia.
8. Squeeze the labia with your fingers.
9. Lube up your fingers and rub them along the outside of the vaginal lips.
10. Move your fingers over the top of the labia.
11. Grab one of the vaginal lips and massage it by moving your fingers along it.
12. Put your hand on the vulva and just run it through your fingers.
13. Grab both vaginal lips between your index finger and thumb and move them along the lips, occasionally squeezing them.
14. Slide a finger into the vagina, and with the help of your partner try to locate the G-spot. Your woman should switch positions to help the search.

Oral massage on women is described in the following chapter.

CHAPTER 17

The Art of Cunnilingus

A unique kind of touch is the contact of the lips and tongue with the intimate body parts of another person.

Oral massage is a type of stimulation of a partner's intimate body parts with the use of the tongue, lips, or teeth. This practice is becoming more and more popular among men as well as women. Making love with the use of lips is yet another method of giving pleasure which also increases arousal and intimacy. This area of sex is unusually pleasurable but is too often rejected by women. This is one of the reasons prostitutes are in demand. So it is worth paying attention to this subject. Start with imagining sex with the use of lips. Imagine kissing and licking your partner and your partner taking care of you in a similar way.

There are different motives for having oral sex. The interest with new forms of sex, curiosity, experiencing new sensations, taking pleasure in this type of physical contact, or helping a partner get an erection are just some of the many reasons. When it comes to the last example, oral massage has a medicinal application. It helps get rid of a specific ailment. It can also help women who have problems with orgasms. Furthermore, this form of intimate play is irreplaceable when a woman does not want to engage in classical intercourse because of a concern about getting pregnant, or for any other reason she cannot or does not want to have sex.

Cunnilingus, or the licking of the clitoris along with the vagina, and fellatio, which is the oral stimulation of the penis, are important and integral elements of intimate games. Women who want to drive their men crazy should master the art of fellatio. Just after a few tries most women consider this to be extremely satisfying and highly arousing.

Cleopatra, who lived in the first century BC, was one of the most famous lovers of the ancient world. In addition to being extraordinarily beautiful, she knew and practiced oral massage. She was a specialist when it came to fellatio, which delighted her lovers. It is thought that she used this skill for political gains.**(14)**

Side note

Fewer men than women have a problem with oral sex—and not just being on the receiving end of it but performing it. Most men admit that cunnilingus is a source of strong sexual stimuli. But how does one go about cunnilingus?

Female oral massage (a guide for men)

There is no doubt that the clitoris plays a key role in cunnilingus; after all, it is the female counterpart of the penis. Skillful oral stimulation of the clitoris is a guaranteed way to bring a woman to ecstasy. The tongue is a lot more delicate than fingers, which means that stimulating the genitals with it will also be a more delicate form of caressing.

Lesson #1

Begin with gently massaging your woman's entire body to finally focus just on her genitals. It is best if your partner leans against something sturdy, whether in a sitting or lying position, with her legs wide for comfortable access. Relax your neck, chin, lips, and tongue. Slowly start licking her inner thighs and gradually do the same to her outer and inner labia. Then increase the pace a bit and move your tongue smoothly over her clitoris and vaginal opening. Focus on your sensations.

How do you perceive your partner's genitalia? Is such close contact with them a pleasurable experience for you? Try not to rub your tongue too hard against the labia and remember to keep your tongue loose for best results. If you keep your tongue too stiff, it may actually create an unpleasant feeling for your partner. It is very important that you do not use your fingers during this particular exercise because its focus is the sensations created solely between the mouth and the genitals. Do not expect any reactions from your lover. At first, both of you have to get accustomed to the new situation and check what is pleasing to you. Involve your senses in this exercise, your sense of taste and smell. Taste your woman's mucus. If you experience an unpleasant odor, it is sometimes due to a lack of hygiene, although an intimate ailment is also possible, just as the food she's recently eaten can affect odor.

Rarely anything is achieved right away, and the same goes for oral massage. That is why the time spent on it should be gradually increased, as should its intensity. Experiment with different kinds of touch: rub your lips against her genitals, gently suck and lick them. When trying to please your partner, remember that women, unlike men, generally prefer gentler, steady stimulation. Do not assume that your partner gets aroused by the same things you do.

Do not be too ambitious when practicing this exercise. An orgasm is not the goal. The priority here is too overcome any reservations with the genitals and to learn what you and your partner like. This information and experience can be later used during an intimate massage.

Lesson #2

Now you know the basics and have familiarized and acquainted yourself with your lover's body. It is time to make her experience real delight. As you already know, caressing without lubrication may not be very pleasant. Of course you can use your saliva or a lubricant, but keep in mind that the best lubricants are the compliments and intimate kisses that you give your woman. Let her know that you are fully involved in what you are doing, and it will make her feel confident. Start with licking and kissing her pubic mound, her inner thighs, and the lower part of her belly. Then direct your tongue toward her genitals and move it rhythmically over the folds of her lips and clitoris while observing her reactions. Also, try sliding your tongue in and out of her vagina. Many women do not remain indifferent to such caressing. Next, spread the lips, and while still keeping the rhythm move the tip of your tongue over the exposed surface of the clitoris, all the while maintaining eye contact as much as possible.

When it comes to the best positions, at first start with those which ensure comfort and let both of you fully focus on exploring what you feel. The woman should be lying on her back or half sitting on a bed or armchair with her thighs spread wide open. It is also worth trying this on a table, provided that you cover it with something soft for comfort. While sitting on a chair between the woman's legs, the man will have very good and comfortable access to her genitals. This position enables a long lasting stimulation. It is a good position for beginners, provided that the woman does not feel like she is on display, of course. Even if skeptical at first, she will like it with time. When you are ready and you want to spice things up, try different variations of this. For example, when lying down, ask your woman to kneel in front of you and lower herself onto your face. She should lean her hands on a wall for balance and have her thighs as far apart as possible while maintaining comfort. This position allows penetration of all "nooks and crannies." A woman kneeling with her legs spread wide apart and her torso bent over low can prove to be an especially exciting position.

Lesson #3

Oral massage can but does not have to be proceeded by a pleasant, intimate game. It can be started without any introductory preparations. In that case, the situation usually starts in a standing position and after a little bit of time the couple moves to the bedroom. When lying down, a woman makes access to her vagina a lot easier.

When kissing the vaginal opening and simultaneously stimulating the clitoris, you are sure to give your woman a lot of pleasure. She will surely appreciate the fact that you are trying new things with her intimate body parts. Rubbing them with your lips, licking, sucking, spreading, and stretching them are just some of the things you can do to really excite your partner. Pressing your tongue to her clitoris and then gently sucking it with your lips is a very arousing method.

Men often make the mistake of stimulating their partner too hard, probably because they like that kind of stimulation themselves. Therefore, your partner's reactions should be a guide for you. However, sometimes reactions alone are just not enough. So encourage your partner to tell you what excites her the most and what is not pleasant to her.

Explore the clitoris and the surrounding area with your tongue to find the most sensitive spots. Check her reactions to a very fast tongue movement in that area. Sometimes all that is needed is a subtle contact between the lips and the vulva, barely perceptible, yet so intense.

Side note

You know how much pleasure can be derived from "temperature changes." Have a sip of something cold and massage your partner orally and then drink something hot and continue the massage. Such a "thermal shock" can be very pleasing . . .

Tips for men:

- Remember that the labia, or vaginal lips, require a gentle touch. In most women it is the most sensitive and pleasure-inducing area after the clitoris.
- Kiss the labia as you would kiss your woman's lips on her face; use the same techniques.
- Move along (and sometimes across) the lips, occasionally brushing the clitoris with a finger or tongue.
- Combine kissing the clitoris and lips with the stimulation of the buttocks with your hands.
- While using your tongue to stimulate the clitoris, use your middle finger to find and caress the G-spot, which is located on the front wall of the vagina.

CHAPTER 18

How to Awaken Desire – Intimate Caressing for Both

Intimate caresses

This is the longest exercise so far—it should last for about an hour. Some sort of lubricant, preferably oil-based, and some knowledge of anatomy, specifically the key parts of the genitals, will be needed. Those parts of female anatomy are the pubic mound, the clitoris, the inner and outer labia, the crotch, and the vaginal opening. When it comes to male anatomy, the important parts of the penis are the glans penis, frenulum of prepuce, shaft, and scrotum.

If need be, have a quick anatomy session together before starting this exercise. I assume that all of you can identify those body parts on yourselves, but you may have some trouble with locating all of them on your partner. To make it all clear:

If you are a woman, sit down and spread your legs. Lubricate your vagina and show your partner where all the parts mentioned above are located. He should explore around to familiarize himself with those parts that are on the inside as well. Let him slide in a finger as you squeeze your Kegel muscle, so that he can feel its location. Then your partner should feel around the vagina to get to know its structure and texture. Help him find the G-spot by guiding his middle finger, palm up, inside you and then having him bend it, as if pointing to the pubic mound. You will probably feel a pleasant sensation, which means that he is touching your G-spot. Your partner may feel a difference in texture of this area compared to the rest of the vagina. It may feel a little rougher. If he moves his finger around the G-spot, he will feel it swollen and pulsating.

If you are a man, sit down and make sure everything is fully visible to your partner. Lube up your hand and walk your partner through the different parts of your genital's anatomy, starting with the shaft of your penis and the tip. If you are not circumcised, show her how to retract the foreskin over the crown of the glans penis. More importantly, show her how to stretch it back over the tip. Doing this will be harder if you are erect. So, try it when you are soft. Do not forget to familiarize your partner with the frenulum. Now, all you have left to show her is the "holy spot," also known by some as the "million-dollar spot" or the male G-spot (mentioned in Chapter 5).

Now that you know each other's intimate anatomy, you can start the exercise. It only gets more fun from here.

Where to start?

Begin by slowly caressing each other's fronts as you have done in the previous exercises, not to arouse your partner but for your own enjoyment. Just like before, remember to concentrate, relax and, especially in this case, use a lot of lubrication. Move your fingers over her crotch, labia, and clitoris. Slide a finger inside her vagina. Stroke the Kegel muscle and the walls of the vagina. Then put your finger in deeper and locate the G-spot and caress it until you feel it swell up and pulsate. During this exercise you can sit next to your partner at first, but it is the best if you move between her legs for the rest of the time. This way you will have easy access to her body, and both of you will be able to maintain visual contact with each other.

If the woman is the active one, the situation is similar. Causing an erection is not the goal here. However, if your man gets very aroused and climaxes, it does not mean you should stop the exercise. Just wipe yourselves off and continue as if nothing happened.

Each one of you should take twenty minutes caressing your partner.

This massage can also be performed orally. Oral stimulation is mostly used as an introduction to an intercourse rather than the goal in itself but, in this exercise, focus on sending and receiving the stimuli created in the process. Such training performed regularly will allow you to freely choose a massage technique and come up with your own variations. That will be a proof that you have become advanced in the performance of this art.

If either of you climaxed during the exercise, reward your partner's "dedication" and return the favor.

CHAPTER 19

Erotic Calisthenics for Both Sexes

Erotic calisthenics—what is it?

As the name suggests, it is calisthenics characterized by eroticism. It is supposed to promote general physical fitness but especially sexual prowess.

Erotic calisthenics has its purposes, and that is why the exercises were prepared separately for men and women.

The goals of erotic calisthenics for men:

- Exercising the Kegel muscle—its fitness has a direct effect on the quality of the erection and on the health of the prostate
- Other exercises for better erection
- Decreasing the oversensitivity of the penis, the cause of premature ejaculation
- Increasing the blood flow to the penis, which results in a stronger erection
- Increasing testosterone levels

The goals of erotic calisthenics for women:

- Firming the breasts
- Increasing the sensitivity of the breasts
- Exercising the Kegel muscle:
  - Its fitness has a direct effect on the sensations experienced during intercourse (makes the vagina tighter). Therefore, it affects the ability to have an orgasm.
  - This muscle is responsible for holding in urine. Many women have this problem, especially after childbirth. So only good things come out of exercising this muscle.
  - Prevents the dropping of the uterus

Erotic calisthenics for men include:

I. Exercising the Kegel muscle:

1. Performing the exercise called the "Spring." The vertical spring is performed when the man is lying on his back and has an erection. The woman raises the penis to a vertical position (using her hand or mouth) and then releases the grip. The penis slips out of the hand or mouth and returns to its original position. The object of this game is for the man to squeeze his Kegel muscle as his penis is springing back to its original position before it hits his abdomen. If he is able to prevent it, then the exercise has been performed correctly. It should be repeated in three series of twenty-five times, even several times a day. The length of each contraction should be increased gradually from one to five seconds. Some encourage a length of time reaching even a few minutes.

2. A different variation of the previous exercise can be used, too. This exercise is called the "Sideways spring." During the exercise the man can be standing, sitting, or lying down. The woman bends the member to the side and then lets it go. He squeezes the Kegel muscle

3. Exercising the Kegel can and should be done also with a flaccid member. This exercise can be performed alone or with a partner, but the latter is preferred. She should hold the member and feel the muscle squeeze. By being there and participating in the exercise, a partner encourages a solid training, which only brings real benefits for both.

II. Other exercises for better erection:

1. Bending the penis (not too hard, of course) down and to the sides—when a man is hard and standing up or sitting down on his heels. It is recommended to perform this exercise with the use of the mouth so that the pressure is not too great.

2. While the man is lying down, the woman raises the member to a vertical position, just like during the Kegel exercise. The only difference is the direction of the bending—it should be done toward the knees, which trains the *erection muscles*. When the woman releases the penis from one hand, she catches it with the other right before it hits the abdomen. During this exercise, the Kegel is not used at all.

3. An exercise similar to the one described in the previous point, except that instead of catching the penis with the other hand, the woman lets it drop on her thumb while simultaneously petting the testicles.

4. This exercise involves gently bending the member sideways.

5. This particular exercise is done without a partner. While having an erection, stand up and vigorously move your hips sideways.

III. Decreasing the oversensitivity of the penis, which causes premature ejaculation:

1. When you have an erection, your partner lubricate her hand and make a loose fist, so that her index finger and thumb slightly touch. Next she should put them onto tip of your penis and gently slide them down. Then remove your penis from her hand. Repeat this motion many times. If you are not circumcised, your woman can tighten her grip when you are pulling out to cause the foreskin to get pulled back over the tip. The reason for this is that during intercourse the foreskin stays retracted, so by experiencing stronger stimuli in the form of moving the foreskin over the tip during this exercise, you can gain greater control during sex.

2. Your partner can change the circumference of the "tunnel" created by her hand, which will affect your sensations. She can also squeeze the tip harder on its way in to increase the difficulty of penetration. Maneuvering your penis in or out of your partner's hand is not just fun for both of you; it accustoms you to strong sensations and ultimately allows you to delay an ejaculation.

IV. Increasing the blood flow to the penis:

1. In order to accomplish this goal, the member has to be exercised by squeezing or putting it into some kind of motion. A good blood flow means a good erection; so, it is worth spending some time looking for the right exercise.

Each man is different, so the exercises for this issue will differ as well, from case to case; there is no one solution. However, there are some tips that can help in finding the right exercises:

a. Moving the penis (shaking it, bouncing it, tossing it from hand to hand, gently jerking it, stretching it in different directions, turning in ["doing the propeller"]).

b. Running (can be done in place), but in the nude, so that the penis can move and "jump around"; using a jump rope is also recommended.

c. Kneeling in front of your partner, who should be lying down, and using your flaccid penis. Try to hit your partner's vaginal lips by moving your hips back and forth.

d. Your partner should lube up her hand, grab your penis, and hold it tight. Try to free yourself from her grip without using your hands but moving your hips. This is usually a very good method for increasing blood flow.

V. Increasing the level of testosterone:

1. Raising the penis to a vertical position by pulling the scrotum.
2. Pulling the scrotum in different direction.
3. Twisting the scrotum.
4. Squeezing the scrotum.

Erotic calisthenics for women includes:

I. Exercising the breasts:

1. The appearance of the breasts greatly depends on the condition of the muscles that support them. If these muscles are weak, the breasts droop. It can be reversed by exercising. The exercises recommended to strengthen those muscles are basketball, handball, volleyball and swimming, especially the breast stroke. If you cannot swim, lie on the floor and mimic those moves. Include your partner in this exercise. As you are lying on the floor face down, have your partner sit in front of you in the nude, at such a distance that you will really have to stretch to grab his penis. In this exercise use the freestyle swimming technique instead of the breast stroke, meaning that you stretch one arm in front of you trying to grab your partner's penis, while keeping the other one behind you on your butt or thigh. Then, alternate the hands, by switching their positions. Repeat this exercise often.

2. The breast stroke can also be done with your partner. Position yourselves exactly the way described in the previous exercise, but this time use both hands simultaneously. Stretch them forward to get a hold of your partner's member and then bring them back behind you. Then repeat the same motion. You can also modify this exercise so that you are much closer to your partner and instead of grabbing his penis with your hands, use your mouth. While doing so, put your arms around his torso and then back behind you. You do not have to keep his penis in your mouth all the time, just put it in from time to time.

3. While standing, slightly spread your legs and squeeze your butt and abdominal muscles. Raise your arms to the side to a horizontal position and bring your shoulders back. Hold it for ten seconds, rest and repeat a few more times. Your partner should be standing behind you and holding your breasts.

4. Assume the same position as described above, but with one difference. This time, put your hands together (like during a prayer) and raise them to breast level. Using your shoulder muscles, press your hands together and hold it for five seconds. Repeat this exercise fifteen times. Just like before, your partner should be standing behind you with his hands placed on your breasts.

5. Move your torso to the left and to the right to get your breasts in motion.

6. Ask your partner to stand behind you and massage your breasts using circular movements.

7. Have your partner lie on his back or sit in a prone position; the choice is up to you. Then, lie on top of him so that your breasts are against his body, and slowly move your torso in a circular motion. You can place your breasts on your partner's chest, abdomen, or back.

8. This time do not lie on your man but straddle him instead, in such a way that only your breasts touch him. Move your torso back and forth so that your breasts rub against his body.

II. Exercising the Kegel muscle:

These exercises can be performed in different positions:

- lying down
- sitting on your heels

- kneeling down
- standing up

The following descriptions depict only one position, but you can change them at will or even use multiple ones. It can prove to be an interesting experience because even the slightest change can often bring unexpected results. So, you should experiment, especially since these are very pleasurable experiments. Remember to compare results when using the same position.

1. Lie on your back while your partner puts different objects of varying circumferences into your vagina. He starts with the thinnest object and stops with the one that causes you discomfort when trying to penetrate you. The results should be written down so you can go back to them for future reference when you do this exercise again. The purpose here is to fully relax the Kegel muscle.

2. Assume one of the positions and let your partner slide an object into your vagina (for example, a vibrator, but keep in mind to have it turned off). See how long it takes for that object to slide out on its own. Then put it back in and squeeze your Kegel, trying to keep the object in as long as possible. Write down your results and compare the times it took the object to fall out on its own. This exercise should be done daily over a longer period of time, such as two to three months, and the progress should be monitored by keeping track of the time that you contract your Kegel.

3. The two preceding exercises can be performed with the use of your partner's finger or penis in your vagina. After a while, both of you will notice the difference and you will see how effective it is, even without having to time it.

III. Other exercises

Exercise: when lacking an appetite for sex

Have your partner lie on his back and crouch over him so that your genitals touch. Rub them together for as long as you like. If there is no effect, try it a bit later or the following day. With time, you should notice a difference in how quickly your body reacts to that stimulus. Your appetite for sex should come back soon.

CHAPTER 20

Erotic Games

An animal in the bedroom

What happens in the bedroom should, above all, be a lot of fun, during which no one is tense. Be relaxed, be yourself. Try to shut down your mind and let your instincts take over. Here, in the bedroom with just the two of you, you can really let your primal instincts go.

Here is some advice on how to free your instincts from time to time. Do not have any limitations: lick, suck, gently bite, and make wild animal noises while your partner lies down. It is time to awaken all the things that are buried deep within you. You can change the roles and play around for as long as you want. This exercise has the best effects when done spontaneously.

Caress all the senses

Let's assume the active person in this exercise is the woman. Her goal is to affect her partner's senses, and her own, as well. First, please his sense of sight. Put on something that your lover likes seeing you in. It can be something sexy but preferably nothing too provocative. Make sure you feel comfortable in it. Then take care of his sense of smell: light fragrant candles or incense, or put on some perfume that he really likes. Next, satisfy his sense of taste by preparing a light snack and some wine. Then turn on some romantic music for his sense of hearing. When all is ready, invite your lover to the room you have prepared for him and give his sense of touch a treat as well by performing a massage. An awesome, pleasing massage.

Tasty tips: food as an element of intimate play

Tryptophan is a substance that is transformed into serotonin, which, in turn, affects libido. Pork, chicken, calves' liver, turkey, and other proteins, as well as seeds, nuts, and avocado all contain high levels of tryptophan. Find a recipe incorporating some of these ingredients. Use avocado to make a sauce, which you will pour over the main course—your partner's body.

Intimate massage in the water

Taking a shower or bath together can lead to a very sensual massage, but more importantly it can be loads of fun for the both of you after a long, tiring day. Just the fact that your bodies are already wet guarantees an enjoyable sensory experience.

Water running over the skin has a calming effect. It betters the mood even when you are alone. Those benefits are increased exponentially when your partner joins you. Soap up each other's bodies slowly and sensually. Tenderly stroke the different parts of your partner's body. If you are up for it, exchange oral massages in addition to your "usual" caresses. You might find a terrycloth mitten very useful at this time; when rubbed against the skin it produces a tingling sensation which is very pleasing.

Do not be embarrassed by each other's nudity, just be like kids having a good time. Well, maybe not exactly like kids. Throughout this entire time try to maintain eye contact with each other.

Wiping each other with a towel is yet another opportunity to show each other affection. Vigorous wiping warms up and stimulates, while gently wrapping your partner with a towel relaxes.

A tub of pleasure

There are two kinds of people, those who prefer a shower and those who would never give up their tub for anything. If you are in that second group, try performing an intimate massage in a tub. To make the moment even more enjoyable, you can add fragrant oils to the bath. Also, use foamy soaps and shower gels to make the skin even more slippery.

A large tub is also a great place for a foot massage. You do not have to be an acupressure specialist to do it, just improvise. Massage your lover's neck, shoulders and back. Warm water has a good effect on all muscles of the body. Pay attention to each other's reactions and let them be a guide of how to touch. Washing each other's hair can also bring a lot of pleasure because it can be combined with a head massage. This mundane activity, performed by a loved person, changes into a sensual experience because the head has many nerve endings. So scratch and caress it. After the bath, which unfortunately dries out the skin, it might be a good time for a massage with the use of a moisturizer. The woman should lie on her front first and ask her partner to spread the moisturizer from her toes up to her neck. After that, she should turn around and the man should take care of her front side. He should make sure that she feels like a real star, with her own private masseur—or a masseur-lover, to be more exact. When the relaxing and erotic massages combined with the moisturizing are done, the man should focus on massaging his partner's intimate area. What happens after that is entirely up to you.

A few ideas to try when sharing a bath

- Soap up or let your partner soap up your breasts and then sit behind him. Use your soapy breasts to massage your lover's back. When doing so, reach around and gently caress your partner's genitals.
- Fill the tub with warm water and ask your woman to kneel in it and bend over toward the faucet. She should find something to lean on. Then, get in and kneel behind her. Start massaging her breasts and rubbing your penis against her body. While that is going on, she can use the showerhead to direct a stream of water between her legs, doubling her pleasure.
- Fill the tub with lukewarm water and get in. Take the showerhead and aim the stream at your woman's clitoris. Alternate hot and cold water. The temperature differences cause better blood flow and increase sensitivity to the genitals.
- Get in a bubble bath and sit facing each other. Put your legs on your man's thighs and rub up against his penis. It can be easier to do this if you use the tub's edge for support.

CHAPTER 21

Intimate Exam: Healthy Fun

A man's intimate examination includes:

1. Retracting the foreskin when the penis is flaccid
2. Retracting the foreskin during an erection
   In both cases, the purpose is to check for phimosis, a condition where the foreskin cannot be fully retracted over the glans penis.
3. Checking for any irregularities on the penis, such as swelling, wounds, etc. and if there is any pain during contact
4. Gently and then firmly squeezing along the whole member with the hand.
5. Bending the penis during an erection.
6. Stretching and gentle jerking of the member.
7. Massaging and gentle squeezing the testicles.
8. Checking the size of the testes.
9. Stretching and gentle jerking of the testes.
10. Stretching the scrotum.
11. Examining the crotch and groin.
12. Looking for the male G-spot.

13. Checking how fast an erection is reached.
14. Checking the quality of the erection.
15. Checking how long an erection lasts when all stimulation is stopped.
16. Checking how long an erection lasts with stimulation.
17. Checking how much pre-ejaculation fluid is excreted.
18. Checking the strength of the ejaculation—does the semen shoot out or does it flow out.
19. Checking the amount of semen during an ejaculation.
20. Checking the amount of semen during a second ejaculation following the first one as soon as possible.
21. Checking a man's reaction to:
    a. Stretching his penis once
    b. Squeezing it once
    c. Retracting his foreskin
    d. Holding his balls
    e. Squeezing the base of his penis
22. Checking the amount of orgasms in an hour.
23. Checking how many orgasms during a day.
24. Checking the amount of orgasms during a course of three days (do not go overboard, of course).
25. Discovering how many "springs" (the Kegel muscle exercises) can be done until the loss of erection.

A woman's intimate examination includes:

1. A breast exam—looking for any irregularities: swelling, lumps etc.
    a. while lying down
    b. while standing up
2. Gently squeezing the breasts—the acceptance of stronger stimuli will come with time.
3. Jiggling the breasts (moving the torso from side to side).

4. Checking the breasts' sensitivity to touch.
5. Checking the sensitivity of the nipples to stimulation (stretching, twisting, sucking and pressing them into the body).
6. Checking for any irregularities in the intimate region: the clit, the lips, the vagina.
7. Looking for the G-spot.
8. Checking the amount of mucus.
9. Checking how well the Kegel muscle works:
   a. by squeezing it around your partner's finger (the harder it is to remove the finger, the stronger the Kegel).
   b. by placing an object into the vagina and squeezing the muscle to see if the object remains in there or at least slides out slower. (First check how fast the same object slides out without having the obstacle of a contracted Kegel muscle.)
   c. By squeezing and releasing the Kegel—that is, by putting objects into the vagina and making them slide out
10. Looking for the "holy spot"

Why do these examinations? Well, for two reasons: for fun, and to verify that the exercises contained in this book bring real results. You can also do it to check the effectiveness of different medications, which you may be taking unnecessarily, but be sure to discuss this with your doctor before abruptly stopping any medications.

I mentioned fun first because when you do these check-ups, you should not have to worry that there is something wrong with your partner. Assume that all is right and just have fun with it. That way you are doing it for health's sake. It is also a very useful form of entertainment because if there is something wrong, the faster you find it, the easier it is to treat.

CHAPTER 22

Just for Women: Twenty Two Ways to a "Happy Ending"

1. Classical massage: basic variation. Massage the penis in the traditional way, grabbing it with the thumb just below the tip.
2. Classical massage: inverted variation. The position of the thumb differs from the basic variation. This time grab the member with a thumb at its base.
3. Using one hand massage his penis only in the upward direction, from its base to the tip (the man can be standing, sitting, lying, sitting on his heels, kneeling—I recommend trying all the different positions). One can also grab the penis in four different ways (described under "Massaging the front and back side of the penis" in all these positions, in Chapter 6.
4. Massage in the same direction as described above but this time using both hands.
5. Now massage with one hand in the opposite direction, from the tip to the base (use a lot of lube).

6. This time alternate both hands in the same direction as in point 5.

7. "Rolling the Dough"—place the penis between the palms of your hands and massage it by moving them back and forth as if rolling some dough.

8. The "Roller"—massage the penis using just one palm while the member is pressed against the man's abdomen. (This method works best when lying down, but try out other variations: standing up, sitting, or kneeling. It is worth a try.)

9. The "Spring"—while the man is lying down on his back with an erection, raise the penis to an upright position and let it go, then repeat.

10. An oral massage.

11. A massage of the frenulum with a finger.

12. A massage of the frenulum with the tongue.

13. A massage of the scrotum with an open palm.

14. Raising the member to an upright position by pulling the scrotum.

15. Twisting the scrotum.

16. Shaking the penis while holding it at its base.

17. Pulling the foreskin off and onto the tip with fingers.

18. Twisting the foreskin.

19. Massaging the base of the penis.

20. Massaging the area where the penis and the scrotum meet.

21. The "Throttle"—grab the penis from the outside with one hand (with a thumb either at the base or at the tip, you can also change the position of the hand during the massage). Move your wrist as if you were revving a bike.

22. Squeeze the penis firmly in different spots along the shaft and then do the same thing, using the other hand.

CHAPTER 23

Eastern Wisdom

Erotic tantra. Tantra literally means "the web of life," but it can be interpreted as a specific attitude toward human life, which incorporates the physical as well as the spiritual aspects. Human sexuality in tantric terms is a path of progress, something more than just physicality. It is experiencing sexuality on a deeper, fuller level.

Tantra stresses the importance of the right attitude: one's sexuality is supposed to serve that person, not the other way around. It is a tool to improve the quality of life. When using tantra during intimate encounters, it should not matter whether one gets aroused or reaches an orgasm; instead, enjoying each other's touch and company is what matters.

Tantra teaches that, when it comes to sex, people are the subjects, so one should not worry that something went wrong or that one did not check out as a good lover. Life is sinusoidal in nature. Next time it will be better. It also teaches us to pay more attention to a person's emotional states, along with breathing and thoughts that come to us during sex. It is important to be in a similar mood, which often has to be attained by working on it together. One has to be able to accept that a partner may be in a bad mood or be angry. By opening up to the other person's emotions one can build an intimate mood and oftentimes a few affectionate gestures or a certain way of touching can help to attain that goal more than a long conversation would.

A tantric massage should encompass the whole body, not just the intimate areas, but also the face, abdomen, arms, and legs. These body parts are responsible for the equilibrium of energy in the body, and their skillful stimulation relieves tension and negative emotions. For example, the knees are responsible for a good mood. Caressing them from all sides causes a flow of life energy to the kidneys, which in turn positively affect the condition of one's sexuality. The thighs should be massaged from the bottom up to intensify a partner's sensations.

Exercise: the chakras

A chakra is defined as a place where the energy connects with the outside world. There are seven chakras in the human body and they are located along the spine: at its base, below the navel, in the solar plexus, near the heart, near the throat, between the eyes, and on top of the head. To free the energy locked in those chakras, start the massage at the head and move toward the hips.

The chakra located at the base of the spine contains the psychic energy described as the Kundalini snake. In a state of arousal the snake moves up the spine, stimulating the other chakras. According to tantra, sex is a process culminating in a state of all-embracing bliss more, than an orgasm, which is just its physical manifestation. The lovers' bodies and minds are saturated with ecstasy.

During intercourse, people go through four phases, which are beta, alpha, theta, and delta, respectively. The beta phase is a state of normal consciousness, the alpha phase is a state of relaxation, the theta phase is a state of bliss, and finally the delta phase is a state of utmost fulfillment and unity. The names of the phases have been borrowed from the different stages of sleep, where the delta phase is a state of detachment from reality and a world of dreams. After such an intense experience, it may be hard to return to reality. So, they can just lie there holding each other, looking into each other's eyes as their breathing and heartbeats slowly return to normal.

The Tao of sex

The Tao of sex is simply the Chinese teachings about sexuality. In our Western culture, during sex we strive toward an orgasm and the discharge of sexual energy. It means getting rid of it, but Taoism teaches to cumulate that energy. The love game should help us do that, and with each intimate encounter we should have more vital strength. When large amounts of this life energy have been gathered, the body will be more efficient, less prone to stress, and one will be able to enrich his or her spiritual side. This way sex becomes something much more than just satisfaction from a moment of orgasm. It brings satisfaction for a much longer period of time. It also helps us become better people who are happy with life as we walk down the path of progress.

People may wonder if the techniques suggested by Taoism are not too hard. It is not something we are born with and it requires practice, but the results will not be disappointing. The level of experienced pleasure will be much higher than anything one has known so far. So what is the secret? Well, it is quite simple. Instead of discharging all that sexual energy, stop just before you climax.

When you are just a step away from an orgasm, calm down, both physically and mentally, and try to spread that energy evenly throughout the body. The arousal will lessen a bit and one will still be able to feel pleasure. Not just in the genitals, like in traditional sex, but in the whole body, with more intensity and for a longer period of time. In the long run, it is helpful not only to the body, but to a person's emotions and personality as well.

Following are some exercises that strengthen the lower part of the torso. The places these exercises focus on are responsible for our bodies' vitality, longevity, and positive sexual energy. If one is able to strengthen these places, the energy will easily flow up the spine. They have been mentioned earlier in the book, but in Taoism they play a key role, so here they are again.

Exercising the anal sphincter

This is a basic exercise in Tao philosophy. According to tradition, the age of a person can be determined by the agility of the anal sphincter. Exercising this body part regularly decreases the probability of getting hemorrhoids and improves vital strength and sexual prowess. The basic form of this exercise involves squeezing and relaxing the muscle a dozen or so times a day.

Exercising the crotch muscles

To be more precise, these muscles include the anal sphincter, as well as the muscles at the base of the penis for men and at the entrance of the vagina for women. These muscles cross together at a point called the "holy spot," forming a "figure 8." This point, also known as the "million-dollar spot," prevents genital illnesses and sexual problems. Strengthening the muscles in this area helps men achieve a stronger erection and keeps the prostate in good shape. It also increases the blood flow to women's reproductive organs, which also increases pleasure during sex. In both genders, exercising the crotch muscles causes general relaxation, decreases tension, and stimulates the activity of the endocrine glands.

Squeeze and relax all the crotch muscles a dozen or so times a day.

Exercise: massaging the "holy spot"

This is a relatively delicate place, so it can be massaged, for example, through a material pleasant to the touch. Do it for about two minutes, using circular movements and gently applying pressure. This exercise can be done alone, but it is better with a partner. The process allows the energy stored in the area to flow freely up the spine to the remaining chakras. It also benefits men because it helps keep the prostate healthy.

Exercise: squeezing the vagina

Lie down. Your partner inserts two fingers into your vagina. Then you squeeze and relax your vaginal muscles around them.

The above-mentioned exercises are based on squeezing and releasing the Kegel muscle. For more information on this topic, refer to Chapter 4.

The following exercises help strengthen the sexual energy and help regulate hormones and prevent sexual disorders.

Exercise: breast massage

This exercise awakens vital and sexual energies. Rub your hands together until they become warm, and then place them on your partner's breasts. Massage both breasts simultaneously with the left hand, moving in a clockwise direction. Do this at least thirty times and then switch direction.

Exercise: penis massage

Lubricate your man's penis and use one hand to slide it up and down the member for a while, and then switch hands. Next, using one hand, squeeze the penis in different spots along the shaft a few dozen times and then do the same thing using the other hand. Finally, rub the penis up and down with the open palms of both hands.

CONCLUSION

Intimate and erotic massage: the joy of healing

Intimate massage is still an inadequately appreciated method of fighting many ailments. Perhaps one of the reasons for this is that this form of treatment requires engagement from the patient, in the form of opening up to someone else and trying something new. As we all know, many people avoid any kind of experimentation. They hope prescribed medications restore their health. Receiving traditional treatment helps resolve a physical or a psychological problem. However, there is much more to gain through intimate massage because it provides not only physical pleasure, but it also engages one's spirituality. It has a downright incredible effect on other areas of a person's life.

The mind and body are inseparably connected to one another. When one is not well, the other suffers with it. It also works the other way. When the body is being positively influenced, the psyche is in great shape as well.

Naturally, visiting a masseuse every day may not work out for everybody, but a regular massage may help you forget about a lingering pain or other affliction. During sexual arousal the brain produces "happiness hormones"—endorphins—which have a similar effect to opiates such as morphine or heroine. In order for the endorphins to be released, one must stay aroused for no less than an hour. After that time the mind enters a higher level of consciousness. As the orgasm occurs, the brain releases such an abundance of endorphins that they will be active as a painkiller within the body for at least a few following hours.

But that is by no means the end of the good news. The immune system also benefits from long sexual arousal, helping keep colds and diseases at bay. Who knows, perhaps a regular massage may prove as effective as a flu shot?

Prolonged sexual arousal also stimulates the respiratory system and blood flow throughout the body, resulting in greater lung capacity and improved circulation.

Chronic headaches, circulation problems, ulcers, asthma, skin problems, depression, and sexual maladies, such as premature ejaculation and other erectile dysfunctions, all have a common enemy. That miraculous method for recovery is, of course, the intimate massage.

So what are you waiting for?

GLOSSARY

Corona *of the penis* - it is the widest "ridge" on the glans penis.

Corpus Cavernosum - the Corpus Cavernosum is one of a pair of sponge-like regions of erectile tissue which contain most of the blood in the penis during erection.

Cure - to make somebody healthy again (Oxford Wordpower).

Endorphins - a type of hormone produced in the body that reduces pain. According to B. Keesling its role is much bigger and is responsible for our good mood. It is produced in large amounts during intimate stimulation. It has a very positive effect on a person's well being and this leads, in turn, to the process of self-healing. "Intimate massage therapy" is a colloquial phrase because, in reality, one has to deal with self-treatment through endorphins initiated by intimate massage.

Frenulum of prepuce - it is a fold of skin that fixes the foreskin to the tip of the member. This area is the most sensitive on a man's body.

Heal - to make someone healthy again after they have been ill, especially by using methods other than medicine > example: The body will heal itself if given the chance (Macmillan Dictionary). *Sexual Healing*—this is a title of Barbara Keesling's book.

(Intimate) massage parlor - massage parlors may employ only licensed personal who are entitled to cure. People learning massage on their own, using this publication, cannot expect therapeutic results.

Labium - it is the Latin word for lip. Labia—a part of the female external genitalia, folds at margin of vulva, majora and minora.

Masseuse - a woman whose job is giving people massage (Oxford Wordpower). In the work „masseuse" refers both to licensed staff and amateurs, but amateurs cannot give promises or suggestions about therapeutic effectiveness. **Massage therapist** is a licensed specialist under the medical law but licensing requirements vary from country to country (sometimes also among states of a country).

Patient - in this work, we use the word "patient" as a synonym to "client" because while our types of treatment have nothing to do with practicing medicine, both those that are healthy and unhealthy can benefit from our suggestions.

Prolactin - it is a hormone which has an enormous impact on a woman's health. It also occurs in men and affects testosterone levels, libido and fertility.

Scar - A massage causes better blood supply to an affected area, better nourishing the skin layers which are responsible for renewing scar tissue.

Shaft of the penis - the main part of the penis from the base to the glans.

Specialist - see *Masseuse*

Stem of the penis - see *Shaft*.

Subconsciousness - in the book *Love, Medicines and Miracles* Bernie Siegel, MD describes a case of some women who thanks to meditation caused the enlargement of their breasts. Carl Simonton, MD gives an example of a man who was able to get rid of his impotence by visualizing the process. From *The Secret* by Rhenda Byrne we can find out that studies, conducted in the USA using biofeedback equipment, confirmed that people who imagine themselves running, trigger activity of the same muscles as when they are active in reality.

A massage will not cause an enlargement or firming breasts against woman's will. If she really wants it, a massage helps to affects her psyche and well-being while the "subconscious will do the rest" as Joseph Murphy, PhD the author of *The Power of your subconscious mind* describes.

Taoism - it is a philosophical and religious system teaching how to live longer, happier, healthier, and wiser. ***The Tao of sex*** is the Chinese teachings about sexuality.

69 position - it is a sex positions in which two people align themselves so that each person's mouth is near the other's genitals, simultaneously performing oral sex.

BIBLIOGRAPHY & COMMENTS

1   *Sexual Healing* by Barbara Keesling, PhD
2   The age of consent for sexual activity vary by jurisdiction from country to country. In most European countries the age of consent is 15. Spain has the lowest age of consent(age 13)
3   A massage does not change harmful habits, but thanks to its influence for the body and psyche, can cause a desire to change his life style > *Sexual Healing* by Barbara Keesling, PhD
4   Scientists of *Wilkes University*
5   *Sensual Massage for Couples* by Gordon Inkeles
6   *A Natural History of the Senses* by Diane Ackermann
7   *Sex and the Paranormal* by Paul Chambers
8   *A History of the Modern World* by Paul Johnson
9   *A Natural History of the Senses* by Diane Ackermann
10 For instance, aspirin which improves circulation of blood may cause internal bleeding
11 *North Jersey Mental Health* - organization licensed by New York State
12 As is well-known, drugs can affect people differently. Observing a drugs' effectiveness is essential. If our body, after taking the

prescribed medication does not react for it after definite period of time what for to continue the intake?

13 *Rapport Hite* by Shere Hite
14 *Sexual Secrets of Cleopatra* by Theodore Ransaw